Stem Cell Solutions

The who, what, how, and why of stem cells

by

Dmitry M Arbuck, MD

To my family and friends whose time I borrowed to write this book

Stem Cell Solutions

The who, what, how, and why of stem cells

by

Dmitry M Arbuck, MD

ISBN 978-1-7341237-1-5
1. MEDICINE. 2. HEALTH.

Printed in the United States of America.

Second Edition.

First Printing: October 2019

MANAGING EDITOR
Paul Adams

EDITOR
Matt Jager

COVER & INTERIOR ART
Jay Adams

Warning and Disclaimer

This book is not intended as a substitute for the medical advice of a physician. The reader should regularly consult a physician in matters relating to his or her health and particularly with respect to any symptoms that may require diagnosis or medical attention.

Image Credits

Many images in this book have been donated, these are credited below the image. Other images have been used under license from Shutterstock.com and Vectorstock.com.

Bulk Sales

Please contact us at amei@solucid.com; we will be happy to discuss your bulk purchase needs.

"Surely every medicine is an innovation,

and he that will not apply new remedies must expect new evils."

- Sir Francis Bacon, 1561-1626

TABLE OF CONTENTS

PART FOUR: END MATTER

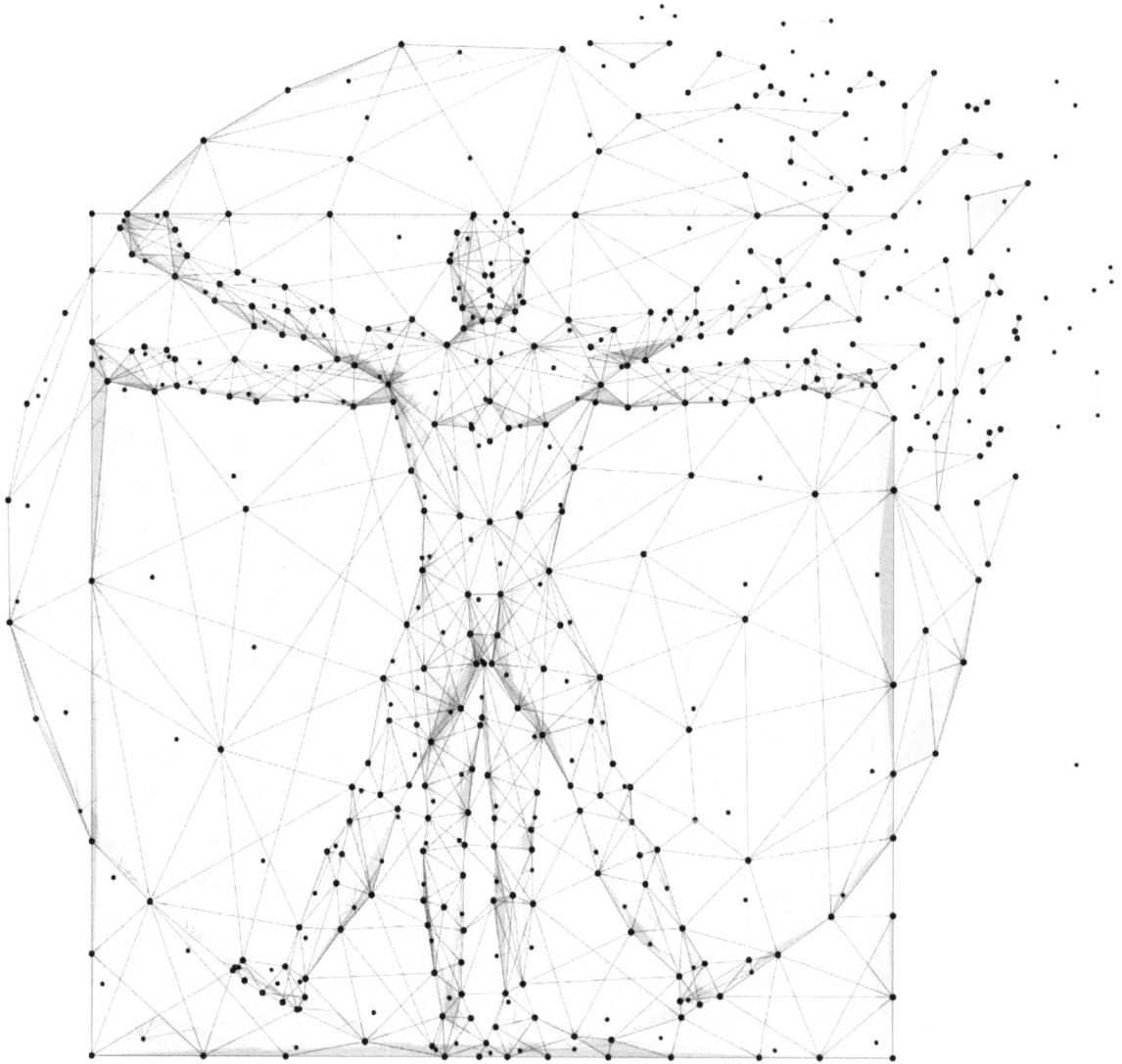

Introduction

You know how it goes: Personal experiences define what we trust and what we apply in our lives. This is especially true with controversial subjects where a commonly accepted opinion does not exist.

Stem cells have intrigued me for a long time. Most pharmaceutical treatments seek to maintain the status quo. We have sophisticated tools to keep blood pressure down, suppress the immune system, control arthritis inflammation, and so on. All of these medications may afford the patient a comfortable life but fail to deliver a cure. With few exceptions, the health care system attends to the symptoms of disease and disorders without eliminating their cause. Stem cell treatments offer a new opportunity: the chance to enhance an efficient self-repair system far beyond the natural capacity of an aging body. What a welcome development!

In the early 2000s, I flew to Germany to learn about stem cells. At that time, stem cell technology was in its infancy. Researchers took questionable paths, working with animal stem cells and human embryonic stem cells, a practice that evoked strong and understandable objections. Stem cells harvested from patients were collected through invasive and sometimes painful procedures. The manipulation of stem cells outside of the body also caused problems. Many of the products labeled as "stem cells" were actually not stem cells at all. If they were, the cells were often dead on arrival.

Clearly, stem cells were not ready for clinical practice in the United States. I returned home, determined to keep an eye on ongoing developments. In 2016, I became aware that several labs in the US had started to offer umbilical cord stem cells. These young, neutral, reportedly safe cells seemed to hold real clinical promise.

The timing was right for me. For two years, I had suffered from a severe auto-immune skin condition. I had an intolerable rash that burned, itched, and constantly left me with painful broken skin. It made my life miserable. I lost 30 pounds and could not sleep. My legs would swell, which made walking painful. I went through the day weak and dizzy. A whole gamut of other non-specific symptoms plagued me. No treatment helped. The only remedy that provided some relief was injections of high dose steroids. At times, the rash covered so much of my body that the nurse had difficulty finding a place to stick a needle.

Without another choice for treatment, I exceeded the annual steroid dose by three times. What else could I do? Oral steroids did not work. Injections provided at most two weeks of relative improvement before the symptoms returned with a vengeance.

Stem cell treatment, which would disrupt my condition at its root cause, seemed the only reasonable solution. No other commonsense approaches were available. At that point, I would have tried anything. I looked into stem cell suppliers. Some, obviously bad actors, set alarm bells ringing. After a thorough vetting process, I identified a lab that offered high-quality umbilical blood stem cells. I made a trip to see the facility and meet the team. I discussed the latest developments with the scientists and saw the actual process of stem cell examination.

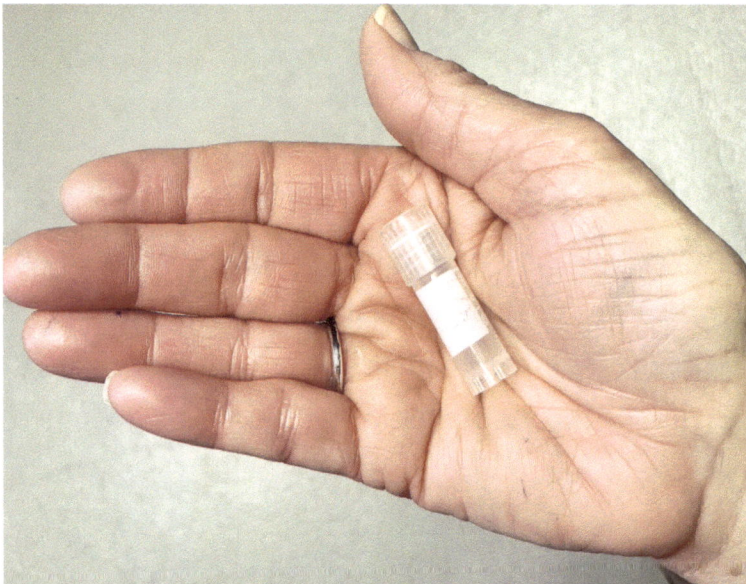

A stem cell vial on my assistant's palm.

Everything seemed to be falling in place. I had a ready patient: myself. I had my otherwise untreatable chronic illness. I had enough knowledge to recognize that, in my case, the benefits of using stem cells likely outweighed the risks.

Understandably, I was anxious. As a physician, I do not want to cause harm to any patient, including myself. Stem cells made sense theoretically, but even the soundest medical theories require the practical grounding of clinical experience. Book learning cannot replace solid clinical judgment. I had to either take a risk by treating my intractable condition with stem cells, or continue hurting myself with the steroids – a known treatment, though ineffective and dangerous in the long run.

The day came. I thawed a frozen cell vial in the palm of my hand.

The contents were infused into my vein. And nothing happened. I felt absolutely nothing. I did not know what that night would bring. Would I have a stroke? Would I turn into some deformed creature? Would I grow a third eye? Fortunately, none of the above. The next day was my day off. That evening, I received a call from Paul, the CEO of my clinic.

He asked how I felt. I shrugged and replied, "I feel nothing." We kept discussing the treatment, and it suddenly occurred to me that I actually *felt nothing*. No burning, no itching. None. Zilch. And my rash was pale.

By the end of the next day, 90% of my rash had disappeared. You can imagine how I felt. If you cannot imagine, I will tell you: It felt really good. Unbelievable, maybe! I had a second treatment two weeks later. After a few days, my rash was about 98% gone. I had an exacerbation in three months. Another treatment took care of my symptoms for six months. Each time my symptoms returned, they were less severe. My fourth and last treatment seemed to take care of my mysterious auto-immune disease, and I am now symptom-free for almost two years. I regained weight and no longer needed to avoid foods, detergents, wool, or any of the other things I had cut out of my life. If my symptoms decide to come back, I know what to do.

In my practice, I treat patients with chronic painful conditions. Many of them have illnesses that do not respond to conventional treatment. My successful self-treatment gave me the courage to offer similar treatments to my patients. I am still surprised by how many remarkable results and otherwise impossible outcomes these unproven therapies deliver. Stem cell treatments have restored the knees, shoulders, necks, and low backs of my long-suffering patients. I have been thanked for the cure of lungs and kidneys, of the gut and auto-immune diseases. I have seen wounds and resistant infections heal, brain function improve, and hearts rid themselves of post-myocardial infarction scars. Many patients, rescued from chronic pain, got off their daily medications and returned to a fulfilling life.

Yes, umbilical cord wall and umbilical cord blood stem cells are still a novelty. There is much more work to be done before they are widely adopted for clinical use. Hidden dangers may later surface. But for patients who have exhausted conventional treatments for otherwise incurable conditions, an alternative is now available.

Throughout history, breakthrough health care technologies – immunizations, antiseptics, antibiotics, aspirin, EKG, MRI, and so on – have transformed the practice of medicine and bettered the lives of millions.

Today, we stand on the doorstep of the next medical revolution: stem cells.

WHO IS THIS BOOK FOR?

When I set out to explore the potential of stem cell treatment over 15 years ago, there was no practical handbook on stem cells for clinicians and their patients. As I write this book, the same remains true today.

Several years ago, I put together a continuing medical education (CME) presentation about stem cells. The goal was to introduce medical providers to the clinical promise of stem cell treatments. The course included a PowerPoint presentation that formed the basis for this book. I hope *Stem Cell Solutions* helps clinicians see clearly the risk and reward of bringing stem cell treatments into their practice. Likewise, I hope this book will improve the scientific literacy of patients seeking relief from intractable health problems, and give them the tools they need to discern stem cell hucksters – of which there are many – from honest health care practitioners.

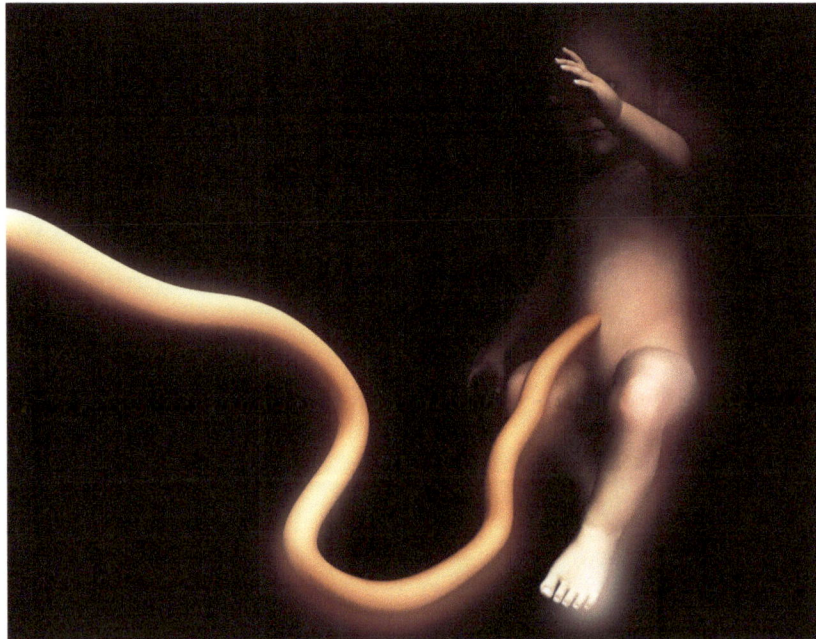

Umbilical cord stem cells come from the umbilical cord and other birth waste donated by healthy mothers after c-section childbirth.

PART ONE:

WHAT ARE STEM CELLS?

Almost all tissues in the body contain stem cell populations. Stem cells may be considered the architects of every other cell. As such, they have the power to repair or rebuild damaged tissue. Successive generations of researchers and clinicians have undertaken the study of how to direct that power.

A BRIEF HISTORY OF STEM CELLS

The term "stammzelle" (German for stem cell) was first used by a German scientist Valentin Häcker in 1868. Following on Häcker's work, in the early 1900's Russian micro-anatomist Alexander Maksimov and others used the term "stem cell" to explain hematopoiesis (how blood cells differentiate into their specialized roles). Through the second half of the twentieth century, researchers discovered stem cells in bone marrow, then umbilical cord blood. In 1981, the developmental biologist Gail Martin isolated stem cells from a mouse embryo at her lab at University of California San Francisco. Since then, the sourcing and harvesting of stem cells have widely diversified, often in response to religious or ethical concerns. Likewise, researchers have explored possible therapeutic applications for everything from autism to sickle cell anemia, from diabetes to auto-immune diseases. By 2017, over a million stem cell transplants have been recorded worldwide. For more data points, see the timeline in Appendix 2, page 61.

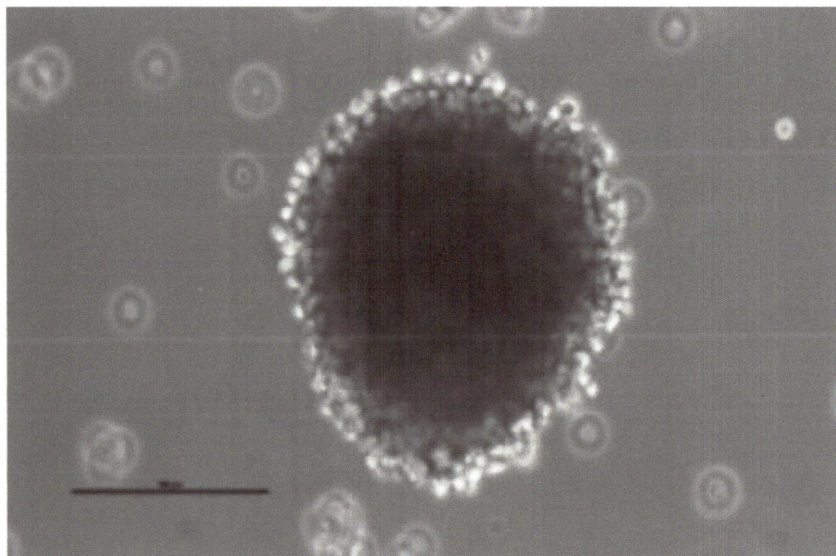

A stem cell 'sphere' that contains hundreds to thousands of stem cells, grown from a single cell.
Courtesy Dr. W. Mark Erwin, University of Toronto

WHAT DO STEM CELLS DO?

In theory, transplanted stem cells should modify inflammation and repair damaged tissue. Although inflammation is a necessary part of healing, unresolved inflammation in the body is catastrophic and, in one way or another, causes the majority of our diseases. Some conditions are broadly recognized as inflammatory: rheumatoid arthritis, asthma, Crohn's disease, inflammatory bowel disease, and cancer. Others are less intuitive, such as obesity or atherosclerosis.[1] In psychiatry, inflammation is associated with psychosis, autism, depression, and others.[2][3][4]

The potential for using stem cells to disrupt the inflammatory process is vast. The immune regulating factors produced by stem cells suppress inflammation and mobilize cells to the site of action. Although stem cell action is hypothesized to direct "healthy" inflammation where repair may occur in a more organized fashion, much remains to be determined.

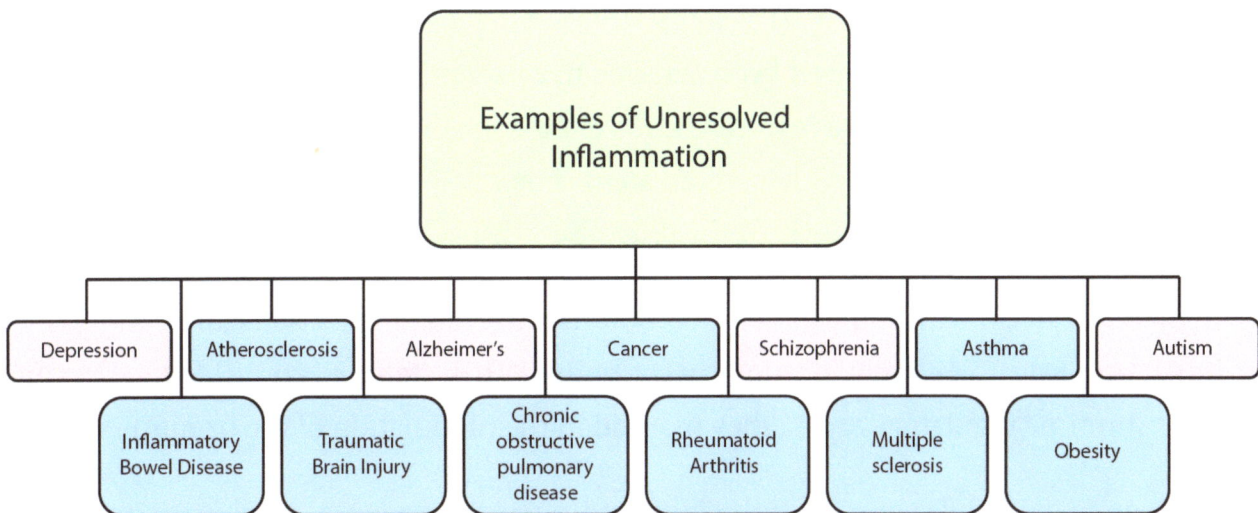

Unresolved inflammation plays a role in many medical, surgical and psychiatric conditions

In addition, stem cells produce cytokines and growth factors, delivered by exosomes, that are involved in wound, heart, bone, nervous system, and other tissue healing (see "Exosomes," page 25). Stem cells themselves are capable of changing their surroundings by immediate physical cell-to-cell interaction. This cellular repair occurs through various mechanisms. Although the full spectrum of stem cells' curative properties likely remains unknown, there is evidence to show that stem cells heal through mitochondrial transfer, direct oxygen transmission from blood vessels to the tissues, and by replacing damaged cells with healthy ones. These and other interactions, including secreted factors that travel from stem cells to other areas around the body, are explored throughout this text.

The regenerative potential of stem cells suggests the most common immediate clinical application of the future may be surgical, showing benefits before, during, and after surgery.[56]

WHAT HAPPENS TO STEM CELLS IN THE BODY?

Settling stem cells in the desired location within the body is called "homing." After infusion, the cells need to identify where to go, and in which tissue to anchor. They seem to sense tissues and organs in distress. They probably have chemoreceptors that allow them to prioritize the risks to the patient's life. Stem cells will anchor (or "home") at the most urgent complaint. If a person suffers from heart disease as well as a muscle tear, stem cells would likely focus their efforts in the heart. Only when the heart is sufficiently repaired will they switch their attention to a peripheral problem.[78]

Transplanted stem cells have never been detected in a patient's body longer than a few weeks after introduction. Much more research needs to be done to understand the survivability, destination, and influence of transplanted stem cells.

If stem cells are injected peripherally (i.e., a joint), they mostly stay within the joint capsule and, therefore, local within the joint space. Soft tissue (muscle) injections allow more cells to be carried away to different locations in the body. When stem cells travel to the thymus, a major immune regulatory organ, they may aid in the modulation of the immune system.

In addition to the cellular impact on the surrounding tissue, stem cells produce extracellular elements such as trophic factors, cytokines, and growth factors that are available to influence the body within hours of stem cell infusion. This is why the clinical response in the treatment of auto-immune problems may be observed within 24 to 48 hours of treatment, while any potential tissue regeneration would require more time.

STEM CELL LIFE CYCLE

Stem cells may replicate themselves, or they can mature into specialized cells, effectively repairing injured organs. Through *symmetric division*, a stem cell divides into two identical stem cells.

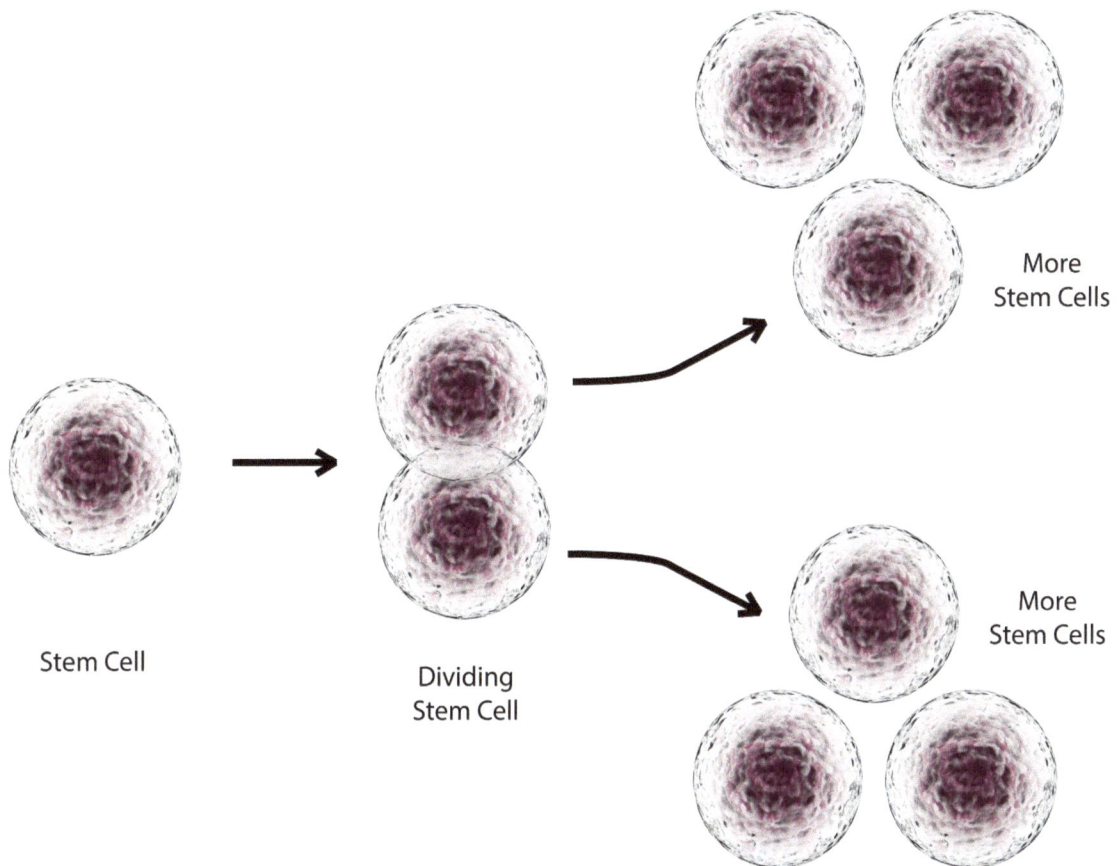

More Stem Cells

More Stem Cells

Stem Cell

Dividing Stem Cell

Symmetric division renders identical stem cells.

Through *asymmetric division*, a stem cell may divide into a copy of itself plus a specialized cell of adjacent tissue.[9] [10] [11] [12] [13]

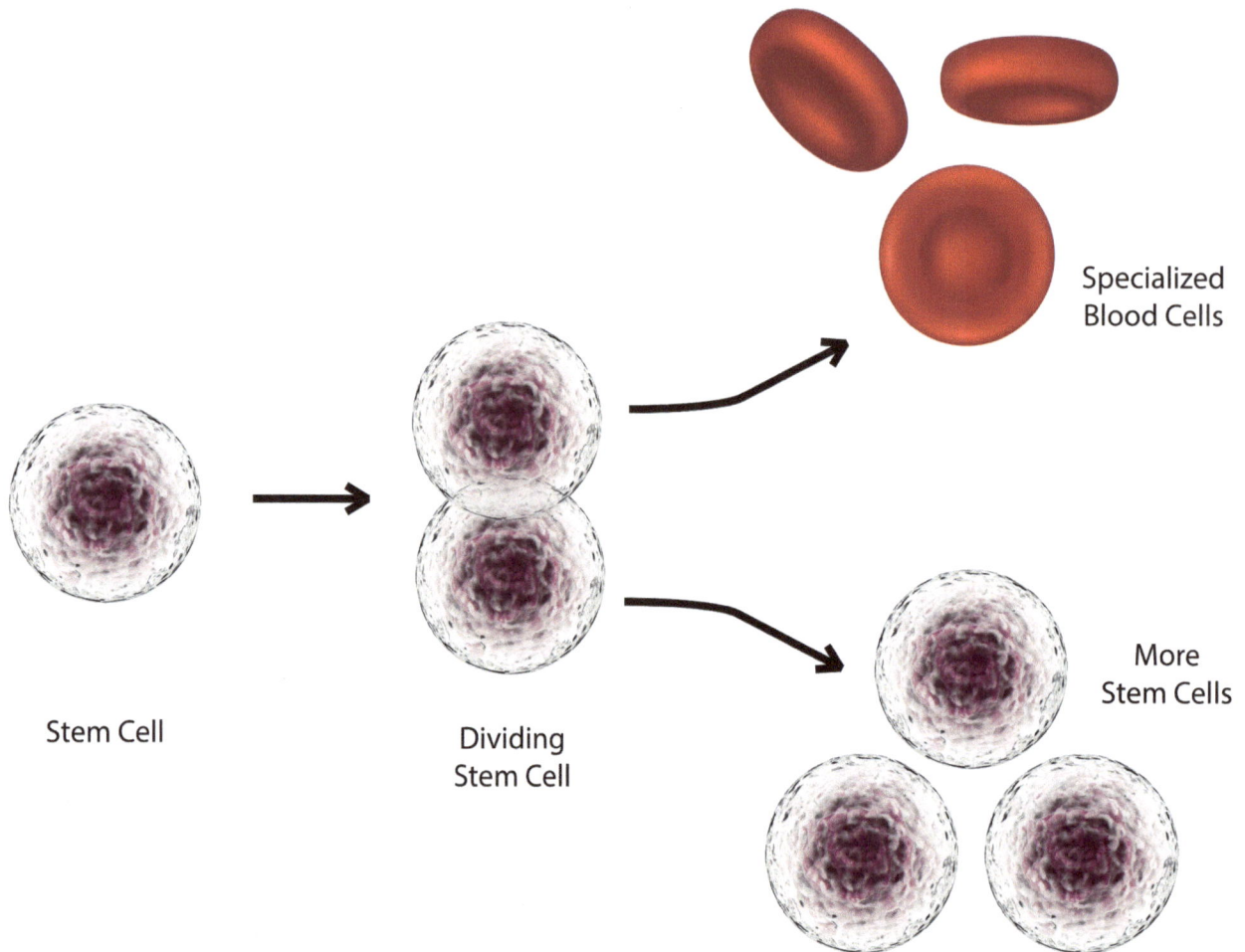

Asymmetric division yields stem cell replicas as well as specialized cells.

In addition to becoming mature tissue, stem cells are capable of reprogramming nearby cells that are sick or damaged by injecting them with healthy mitochondria and other inner cellular parts. This interaction, between a stem cell and a cancer cell, has been observed in a lab environment. Fatigued muscle, heart muscle, endocrine, and nerve tissue may be repaired in the same manner.[14] [15] [16] Whether stem cells consistently reprogram sick and damaged cells through such mitochondrial transfer remains unclear.[17]

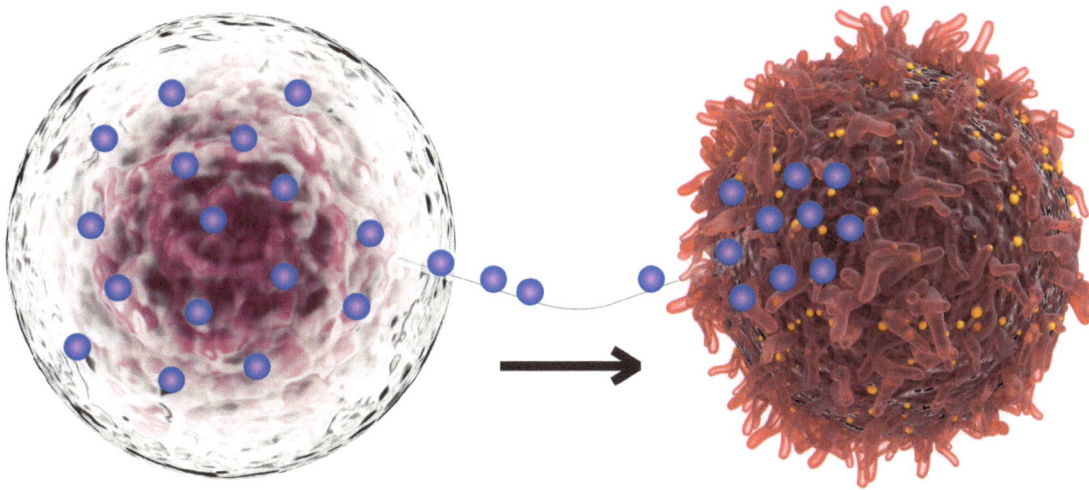

A stem cell delivers healthy mitochondria to a cancer cell.

Stem cells may position themselves on a blood vessel and transmit oxygen and nutrients to the suffering tissue. Even further, stem cells may ultimately form new blood vessels or repair damaged ones. Stem cells love oxygen, but they also increase tissue health by creating a better environment for themselves through the improvement of vascularization.[18][19] This is why introducing stem cells into poorly oxygenated areas of swelling or even into spinal discs may be beneficial.

Some types of stem cells have the capacity to differentiate into nerve cells. One day, we may have the expertise to place stem cells into a damaged brain or a nerve plexus to renew the area with young, new neurons.[20][21] Of course, such treatment remains in the realm of speculation for now.

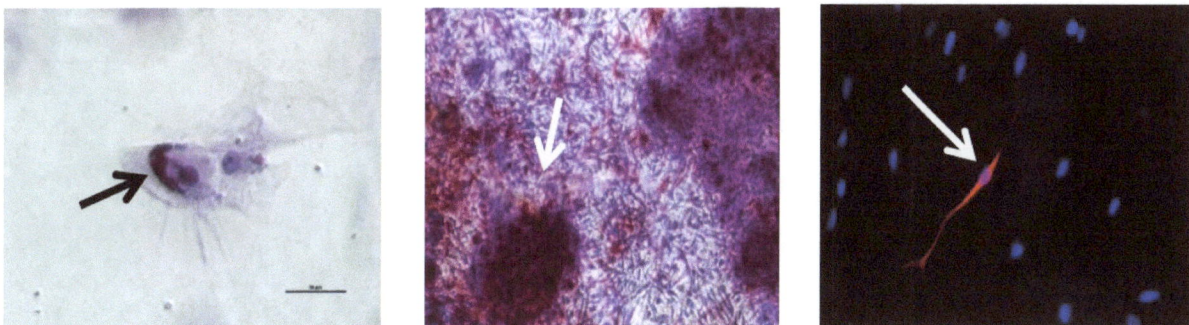

The same line of stem cells differentiated into a fat cell (left), bone cell (middle), and nerve cell (right). Courtesy of Dr. W. Mark Erwin, University of Toronto

CELL HIERARCHY

Stem cells are popularly understood to have the potential to become any cell in the body, but the scientific reality is a bit more subtle. Different types of stem cells possess different potential outcomes. The **totipotent** stem cell, found within the inner cell mass of the blastocyst (the beginning stages of a developing embryo), does have the potential to become any cell in the body. When leveraging totipotent stem cells for medical treatment, their totipotency (literally "potential for everything") can cause problems of indeterminate differentiation. **Progenitor** stem cells, such as mesenchymal and hematopoietic stem cells, turn into a wide but already partly predetermined category of tissues.

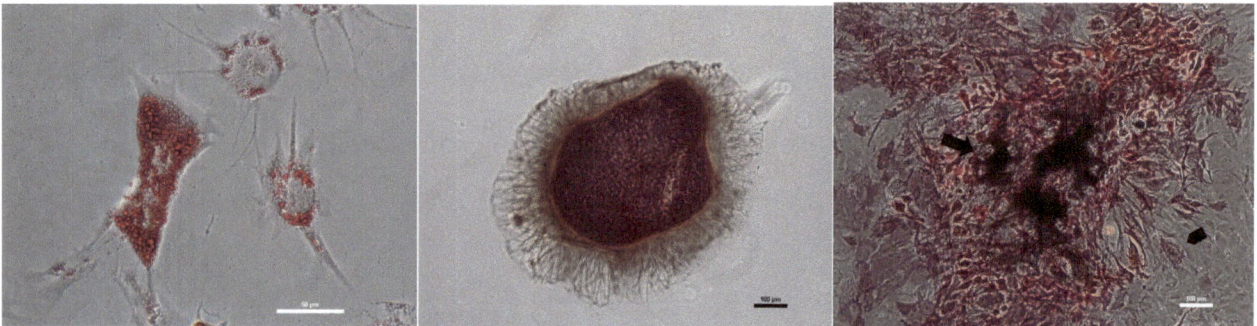

The same line of mesenchymal stem cells produced a fat cell (left), cartilage cell (middle), and bone cell (right). Courtesy of Dr. W. Mark Erwin, University of Toronto

Further maturity gives birth to **precursor** cells that become a line of one or two tissues. Although precursor cells are not quite stem cells and not quite mature cells, in this book, we refer to them as "adult stem cells." Finally, **mature cells** represent specific tissue.[22][23] These four cell types are not absolutely demarcated; there is some overlap in their function.

STEM CELL HIERARCHY	
Totipotent (blastocyst)	Can become any cell or any tissue
Progenitor (umbilical cord stem cells)	Can become almost any cell or tissue with a preference for certain tissue types (i.e., mostly connective tissue with some blood cells)
Precursor (adult stem cells)	Can become a cell or a tissue of a particular type (i.e., ligaments, muscles or cartilage, and not endocrine cells)
Mature (adult cells)	Fully specialized cells (i.e., muscle cells, blood cells, and so on) with no further transformative potential

AUTOLOGOUS AND ALLOGENEIC STEM CELLS

Autologous stem cells come from your own body. They are your own stem cells with developed immune markers. Adult stem cells are a double-edged sword. They are as old as the donor, subject to environmental factors, fewer in number, and less potent (see "Telomeres and aging," page 21). Adult stem cells are more precursor than progenitor cells, and as such, prefer to develop into a

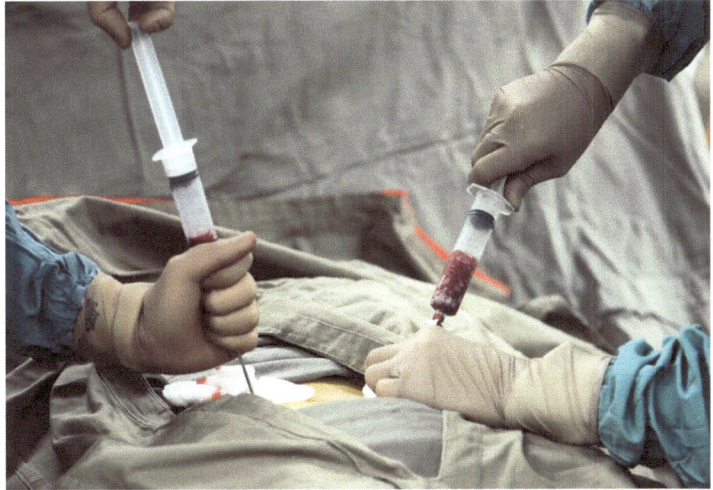

Invasive bone marrow harvesting from a patient

particular type of tissue. Consequently, when transplanted, they may experience aberrant differentiation, including tumorigenesis. In other words, experience shows that your own autologous adult stem cells can sometimes develop into cancer.

Likewise, adult stem cells collected from fat are in fat for a reason: They are more suitable for turning into fat than into any other tissue. Harvesting adult stem cells from bone marrow seems better and more diverse therapeutically, because of the presence of hematopoietic stem cells in addition to mesenchymal stem cells (see "Mesenchymal and hematopoietic stem cells," page 16), but harvesting is more traumatic and expensive.[24][25]

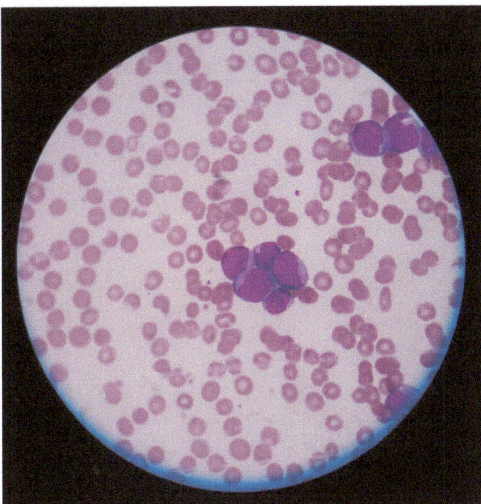

Stem cells in the bone marrow

Allogeneic stem cells come from a donor. If they come from an adult donor, they are **adult allogeneic stem cells** that have already developed immune markers and are commonly seen as foreign by the recipient immune system. This causes auto-immune rejection and the need for active immunosuppression prescribed by the treating physician.

Umbilical cord-derived allogeneic stem cells, on the contrary, are too young to form human leukocyte antigens (HLA), and therefore, they do not possess immune expression. The major histocompatibility complex (MHC) is not developed, making immune conflict with an adult host highly unlikely.[26] As such, when allogeneic umbilical cord stem cells are used clinically, there is no need to test for immune compatibility or to involve the patient in immunosuppression to avoid graft rejection.

Umbilical Cord Stem Cells	Allogeneic Adult Stem Cells	Autologous Adult Stem Cells
Have no immune markers	Have immune markers	Have immune markers
Are not rejected by the recipient's immune system	Likely to be rejected by the recipient's immune system	May be rejected by the recipient's immune system even though the cells come from their own body

In other words, both autologous adult and allogeneic umbilical cord-derived stem cells are likely safe with respect to immune compatibility, with umbilical cells being the safest.

MESENCHYMAL AND HEMATOPOIETIC STEM CELLS

Hematopoietic stem cells are present primarily in blood and bone marrow. They differentiate into blood cells and produce extracellular components overlapping with those secreted by mesenchymal stem cells.

Most current stem cell research is focused on mesenchymal cells. The term "**mesenchymal stem cell**" (MSC) was coined in 1991 by Dr. Arnold Caplan, but its meaning continues to evolve.[27]

Mesenchyme is embryonic connective tissue that is derived from the mesoderm, and that differentiates into hematopoietic

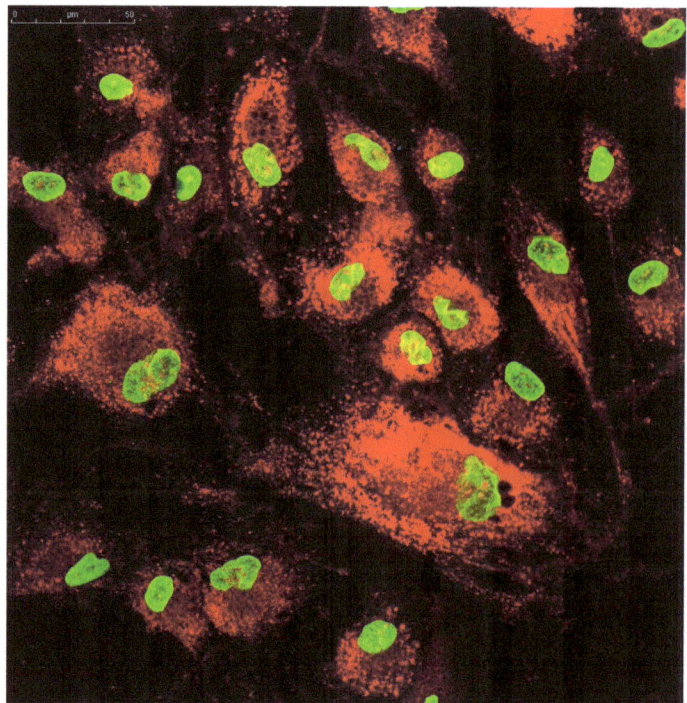

Mesenchymal stem cells labeled with fluorescence molecules.

and connective tissue. Of note, MSCs were once thought not to differentiate into

Fat Tissue

Umbilical Cord

Bone Marrow

Stem Cell

CD105

CD90

CD73

Expressed

CD14

HLA-DR · CD11b

CD31 · CD34

CD79a · CD45

Not Expressed

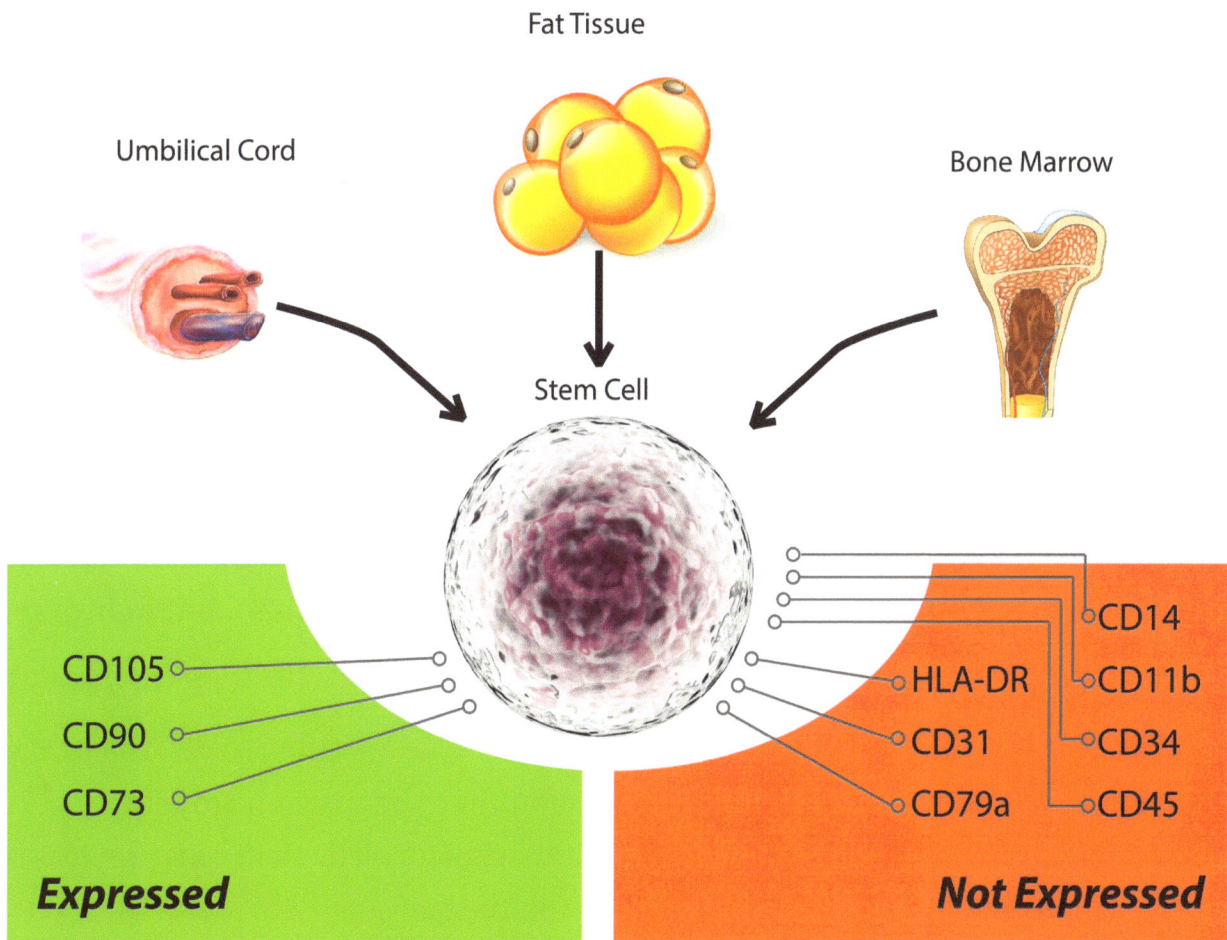

The scientific definition of stem cells comes from a set of specific factors a cell does or does not possess. It is impossible to visually identify a stem cell as it does not look any different from other cells.

hematopoietic cells. The definition of mesenchymal stem cells has recently changed, as they are now known to produce more tissue types than was originally believed. The current definition is based on the presence or absence of specific molecules on the surface of the cell and other factors (see table below).[28]

Current Scientific Definition of Mesenchymal Stem Cells (3, 4)
• Are plastic-adherent when maintained in standard culture conditions
• Express the cell surface markers CD105, CD73, and CD90
• They lack expression of CD45, CD34, CD14 or CD11b, CD79 or CD19, and HLA-DR
• Differentiate to osteoblasts, adipocytes, and chondroblasts in vitro

Mesenchymal stem cells may come from anywhere in the body – not only from the umbilical cord. In this case, they are called *autologous* mesenchymal cells. They are primarily harvested from bone marrow[29] and adipose (fat) tissue.[30][31][32] The umbilical cord wall houses a particularly large population of mesenchymal stem cells.

Adult stem cells derived from adipose tissue will recruit other cells to be more effective within the target niche (the area in need of repair.) Bone marrow stem cells are even more effective at recruiting other cells because marrow contains both hematopoietic and mesenchymal cells. Umbilical cord stem cells, by virtue of their youth, are expected to be even more potent and efficient, though this has yet to be scientifically confirmed.

All stem cell preparations contain a variety of cells. At present, it is technologically impossible to have a sample with 100% mesenchymal stem cells. The difference is the proportion of cells in a sample. Hematopoietic stem cells differentiate into white and red blood cells and plasma components which aid the immune system. Lymphocytes, monocytes, and macrophages also come out of this cell line, aiding in anti-inflammatory processes in the body. As mentioned earlier, mesenchymal cells differentiate into connective tissue and are involved in organ repair. Hematopoietic cells do not form scaffolding, which may explain why they are, to some degree, less effective in tissue and organ repair but likely more potent in immune regulation.

Different stem cell products significantly overlap in their mechanism of action and applications. A combination of mesenchymal and hematopoietic stem cells provides the most balanced and all-encompassing influence on the body.

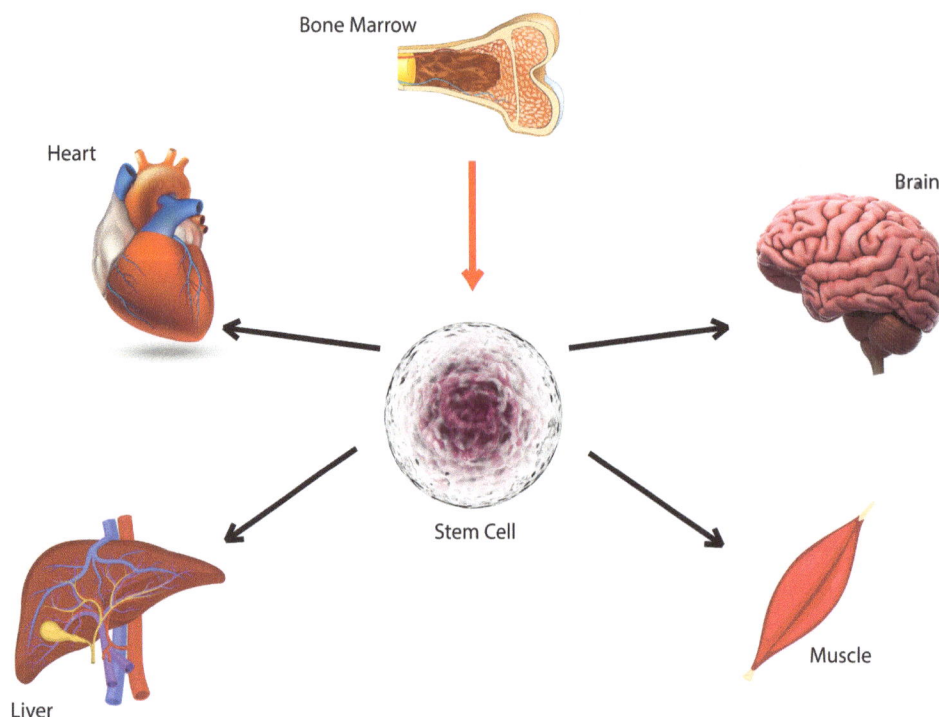

Stem cells harvested from bone marrow may mature into specialized tissue cells, depending on where the stem cells are placed.

FETAL WOUND HEALING

Newborns are, as a rule, healthier than adults. Why? Because during fetal development, active stem cells continuously repair their tissue.

In the 1980s, surgeons observed that after intrauterine surgeries (surgery performed on a baby before birth), babies were born with remarkably limited deformities. Fetal healing occurs rapidly and with minimal scar formation. Using umbilical cord cells for the treatment of adult wounds, therefore, holds major promise.

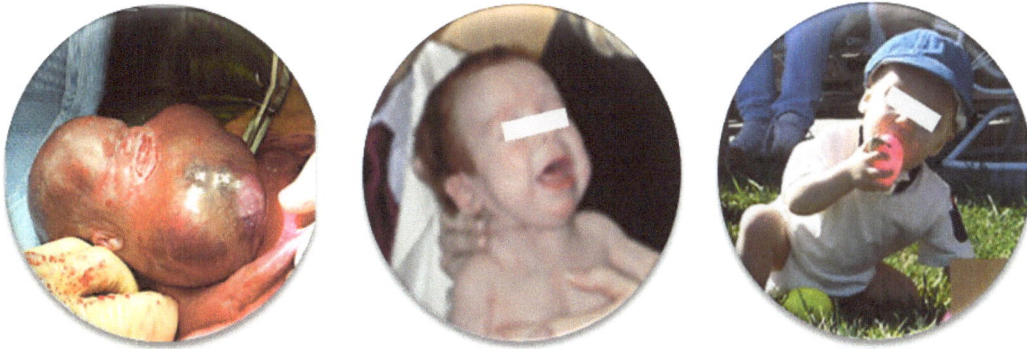

Intrauterine surgery to remove disfiguring facial tumor from a fetus (left). The same baby at birth (middle) and as a healthy toddler with minimal to no scarring (right). Courtesy Dr. Michael Harrison, Univ of California, San Francisco

The amniotic membrane is, in itself, an active organ, and it increases the potency of the adjacent stem cells. Seeding the amniotic membrane with umbilical cord cells multiplies the healing property of both.

We are made of stem cell composite, so to speak, when we enter life. As we age, the number of stem cells drops precipitously. In old age, we hardly have any. It is estimated that just one out of every two million body cells is a stem cell by age 80. Harvesting stem cells from an older donor for autologous treatment is a chore. There are fewer stem cells, and even those possess a limited regenerative ability.

AMNIOTIC AND UMBILICAL STEM CELL PRODUCTS

The birth waste of a healthy newborn provides an ample source of stem cells. These products are *not* sourced from aborted fetuses. The use of embryonic stem cells is strictly prohibited in the United States (see "Embryonic stem cells," page 31).

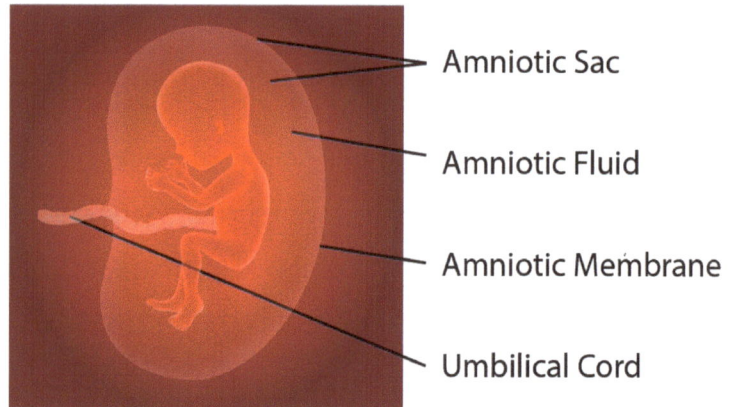

- Amniotic Sac
- Amniotic Fluid
- Amniotic Membrane
- Umbilical Cord

Amniotic fluid (the liquid that cushions a growing fetus) practically lacks live stem cells but is rich with cytokines and growth factors produced by stem cells. There are amniotic fluid-derived products on the market. They have a higher concentration of active factors but produce only local, time-limited connective tissue repair and do not seem to repair the immune system.[33]

The **amniotic membrane** (the lining of the embryonic sack) is covered with stem cells and may be used topically as a healing barrier treatment for burns, wounds, or spina bifida, to give a few examples.[34] However, understanding the practical uses of viable stem cells from the amniotic membrane will require much more investigation.

Wharton's jelly (**umbilical cord wall**) stem cells are mostly mesenchymal cells that are especially suitable for becoming connective tissue. **Umbilical cord blood** stem cells are mostly hematopoietic cells that are especially suitable for becoming blood cells and immune regulators.

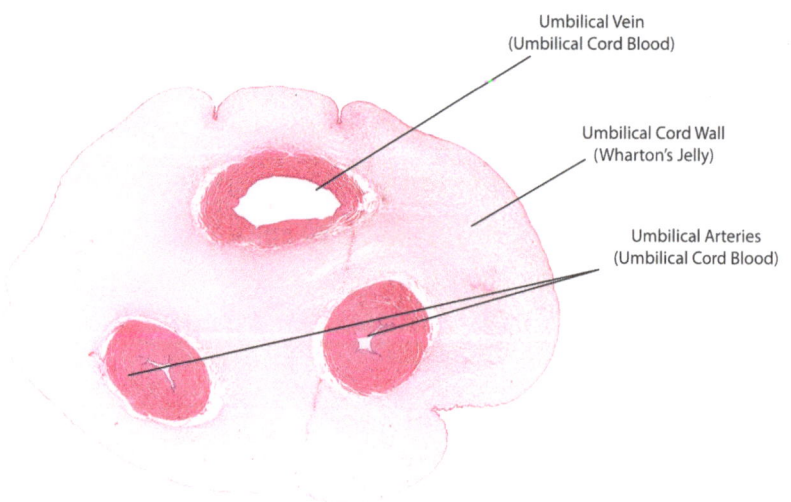

Umbilical Vein
(Umbilical Cord Blood)

Umbilical Cord Wall
(Wharton's Jelly)

Umbilical Arteries
(Umbilical Cord Blood)

This umbilical cord cross-section shows several sources of umbilical stem cells. The vein (top) carries oxygenated umbilical cord blood from mother to embryo. The arteries (bottom left and right) carry blood from the embryo back to the placenta.

Umbilical cord blood and umbilical cord wall-derived products have been shown to be the most promising and safest stem cells for human clinical use. Because of their higher activity, it is expected that transplanted umbilical cord stem cells may actually increase the vitality of adult stem cells already present in the recipient's body. Both mesenchymal and hematopoietic cells are more prevalent in the umbilical cord than elsewhere.[35][36]

Furthermore, umbilical cord blood and Wharton's jelly stem cells have so far not been reported to induce neoplasia (cancer). We can estimate cancer risk by the likelihood of spontaneous cell mutations. By making stem cells immortal in a lab and allowing them to divide endlessly, a Harvard study showed that the first cancer mutation was observed after 1 million divisions. This suggests the likelihood of umbilical cord blood stem cells turning cancerous is extremely remote.[37]

	Umbilical Cord Stem Cells		Adult Stem Cells		Embryonic Stem Cells
	Umbilical cord wall Wharton's Jelly	Umbilical cord blood	Adult autologous stem cells	Adult allogeneic stem cells	
Immune Response	-	-	+	++	+
Oncogenesis Risk	-/?	-/?	+	++	++
Composition of Cells	Mostly Mesenchymal	Mostly Hematopoietic	Mixed depending on harvest site	Mixed depending on harvest site	Mostly Mesenchymal
Risk of Uncertain Differentiation	+	+	++	+++	+++

TELOMERES AND AGING

Telomeres are the caps on the ends of chromosomes that prevent the chromosomes from fraying or falling apart. Without those caps, chromosomes are unstable. Uncapped chromosomes unwind and disintegrate, or fuse with adjacent chromosomes, causing cell death.

TELOMERE

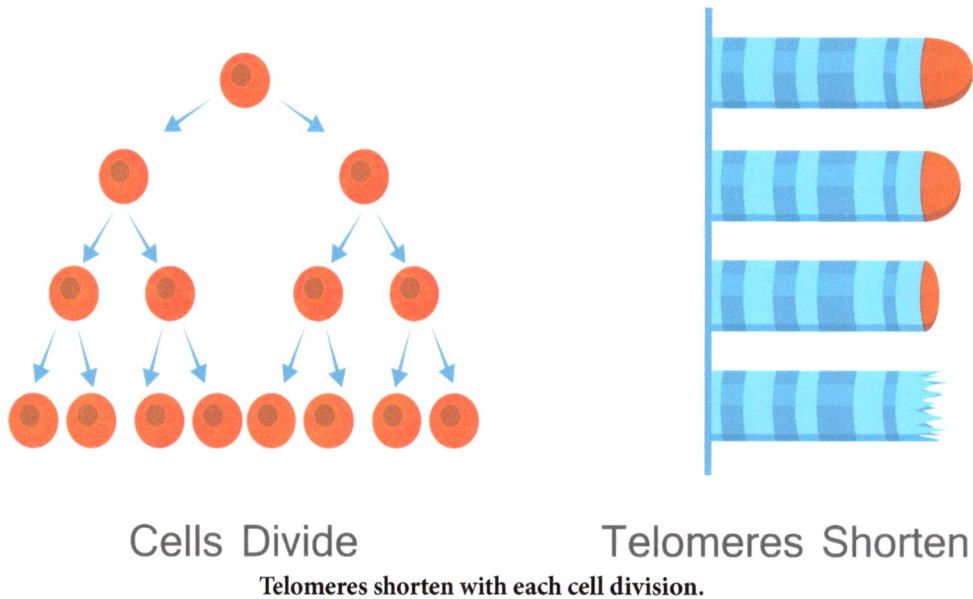

Cells Divide   Telomeres Shorten

Telomeres shorten with each cell division.

Every time cells divide, the telomeres shorten. This is why we age; this is why our tissues get older.[38] We are born with about eight thousand base telomeres and have ten times fewer when we die from old age.

Umbilical cord stem cells have the maximum length telomeres. When they reproduce and repair adult tissue, they donate younger chromosomes, rejuvenating adult tissue.[39][40] This is a source of optimism for regenerative medicine: With regular stem cell treatment, the body is not only rejuvenated – it likely ages slower.

Adult tissue stem cells have short telomeres, and as such, may be active in repairing but not in rejuvenation – but of course, old stem cells with shorter telomeres are still better than fully matured adult cells.[41]

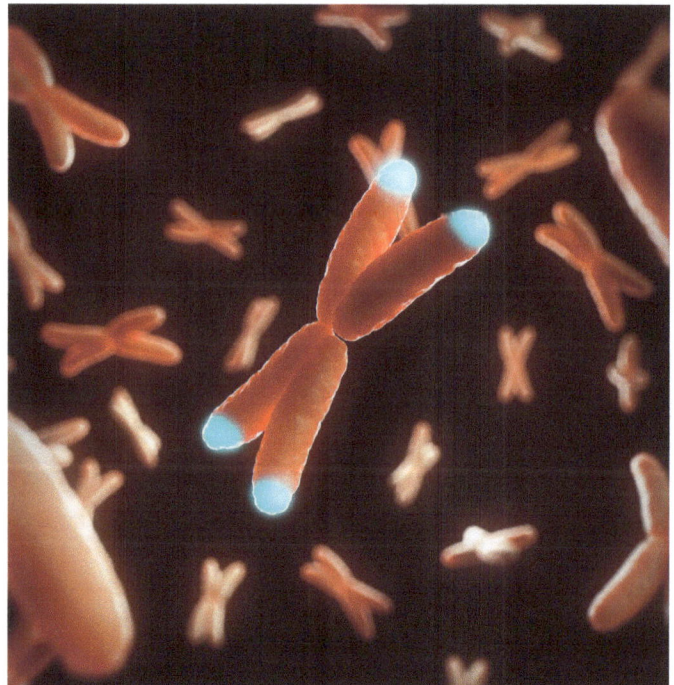

Telomeres are depicted here as blue caps on the ends of the chromosomal arms.

Aging stem cells enter a state called **"senescence."** Such cells retain stem cell function but stop dividing. By mid-age, a majority of stem cells lose the ability to divide, although they continue to repair. This is why the number of stem cells dwindles, and aging accelerates.[42] [43] This is yet another reason adult stem cells cannot fully compete with umbilical cord cells.

Aging stem cells also suffer from mitochondrial dysfunction, which means the cell powerhouses – mitochondria – work less and less efficiently as we age. Umbilical cord cells normally do not share that problem.

In a lab setting, stem cells have been observed to divide approximately every 28 hours and about 70 times. This division cannot be reliably shown in a live organism. The replication rate is variable between species. In humans, multiplication is reported to be as fast as a few hours and as slow as every 40 weeks. This is why original infused cells theoretically may be present in the body for up to three to six months or more. Unlike adult tissue, which has been exposed to radiation, toxins, and mutations, the DNA of umbilical stem cells is young and transposes these features onto the host in which they find a new life.

However, the long-term preservation of whole umbilical cord or cord blood may be technically difficult, and there is no guarantee that cells survive the process (see "Vitality and preservation," page 37). Also, many years of paying for storage may not be cost-effective.

Cellular and extracellular products

Stem cells are largely dormant until activated to multiply, propagate, and influence surrounding tissues. These activities include migrating within damaged organs and healing through both physical contact and secretory function.

The migration of stem cells within the body is a complex and controversial subject, bound up with the question of how stem cells respond to damaged cells and tissues (see also "Intramuscular injections," page 47). Stem cells may repair by their proximity to other cells, in which case they must remain in physical contact with the damaged cells, or by secreting extracellular components that spread around the body and work remotely from the stem cell. The extracellular component of stem cells ("**matrix**") can be collected, preserved, and used clinically for tissue repair. The effect of matrix products is time-limited and is mostly local. The term "stem cell matrix" lacks a precise definition and usually refers to an assembly of cytokines and growth factors derived from stem cells with no actual live stem cells in the composition.

Platelet-rich plasma (PRP) is an example of such a product. It is not a stem cell matrix per se; it is the activated expression of a host of growth factors secreted by platelets that, in turn, act upon the tissue target, such as tendon or ligament. PRP is commonly used because it contains fairly concentrated extracellular ingredients such as growth factors, cytokines, and trophic factors, that come from adult platelets; as such, it can facilitate healing and promote the activity of the native stem cells in the surrounding tissues.[44][45][46][47]

Platelet-rich plasma

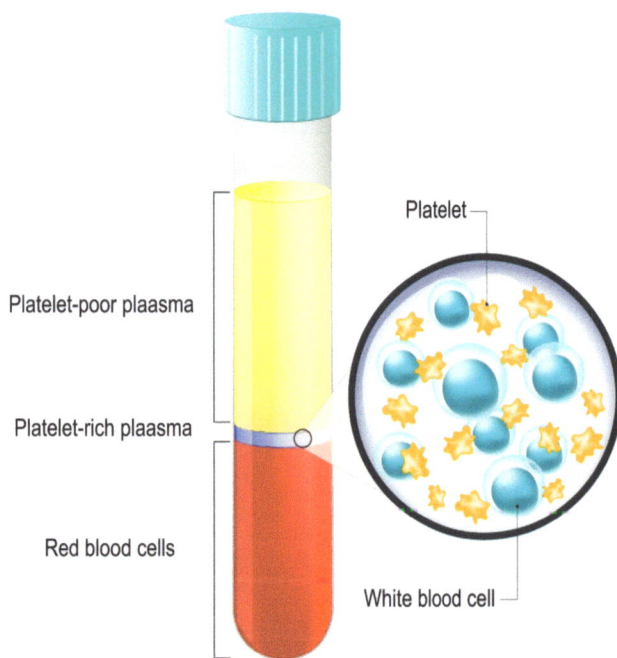

Platelet-poor plaasma

Platelet-rich plaasma

Red blood cells

Platelet

White blood cell

PRP is a fraction of a blood sample.

Some see PRP as a type of prolotherapy with the potential to strengthen tissues by forming new connective tissue fibers and possibly enhancing the properties of existing ones. Like amniotic fluid-derived products, PRP does not repair the immune system but may produce local connective tissue repair that lasts for a limited time. Depending on the location, a positive function of PRP might be the secondary induction of stem cells located near the injection site. In other words, PRP may induce native stem cells to work better.

On the contrary, a recent paper reports that PRP delivered *in vivo* (to a live organism) is unlikely to activate endogenous stem cells and enhance MSC-mediated hyaline cartilage formation.[48] While the study limited its investigation to the effect of PRP on cartilage formation, the findings add to the controversy surrounding various claims about the utility of PRP – which type of collagen develops, the proteins involved, and so forth. In summary, much remains to be determined about both the mechanism and the outcome of PRP treatment. This kind of therapy does involve significant inflammation and the potential of undesirable long-term consequences of scarring.

PRP may be made from umbilical cord blood as well as the patient's own blood. Donors with hormonal challenges, morbidities, and post-menopausal women are thought to have PRP that is less stimulatory.

One study found the addition of even 0.1% of umbilical cord PRP to autologous adult PRP produces a disproportionate, many-fold increase in potency, which testifies to the higher biological activity of young tissue versus mature tissue.[49] The umbilical cord cytokine concentration far exceeds that of an adult PRP. Some factors, such as tumor necrosis alpha, appear to be absent from PRP. This may, in part, explain the higher therapeutic potency of live stem cell treatment. Although one must be wary of drawing far-reaching conclusions from a single study, it makes intuitive sense that the vigor of youth would enhance stem cell products.

EXOSOMES

All tissue cells, including stem cells, contain **exosomes**, packaged payloads of growth factors, cytokines, and other factors destined for secretion from the cell. Nearly all good stem cell preparations will be a primitive source of exosomes in varying degrees of health and integrity.

Exosomes are one of the many components of cellular life – and a relatively simple one. A cell is encircled by a cell wall which surrounds multiple intracellular organs such as mitochondria, ribosomes, and other structures and features. Exosomes are cellular sub-compartments of a living cell, much as cubicles are a part of an office. The Latin "exo" means "outside," so exosomes are defined by their journeys outside of the cell into the outer space of biology for signaling, consumption, or waste disposal. Other similar cellular compartments never leave the cell and are more or less distinguished along lines of function, such as vacuoles, lysosomes, and more.

Like satellites, exosomes can deliver signals to surrounding cells and tissues. These signals are like a bullhorn that calls the rest of the micro-universe to attention – to march, fire, farm, or die. Some direct downstream events are amplified, and amplification, likely, is the purpose of these signals.

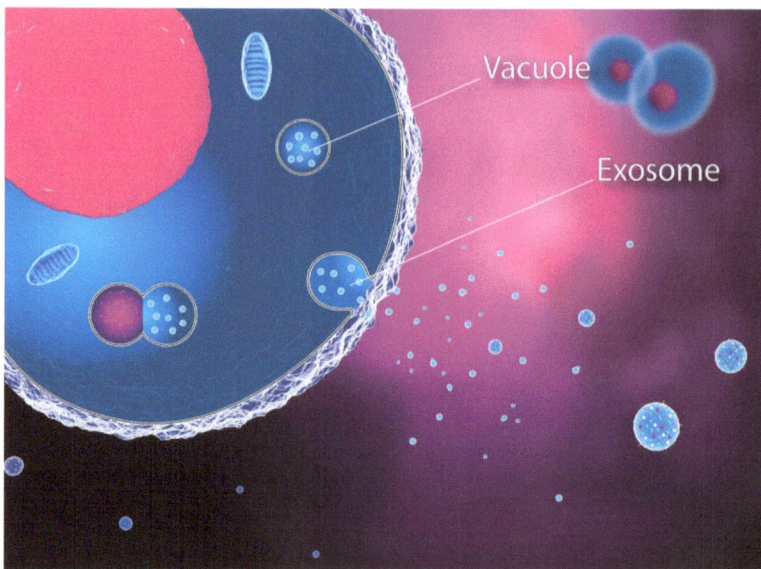

Vacuoles become exosomes when they empty their contents into the extracellular environment.

Exosomes can also be secreted with raw materials or "food" for the benefit of a greater layer: a tissue, an organ, an organism. As for waste disposal, exosomes are garbage trucks, without which we would suffocate in our own waste.

What if exosome functions could be controlled? What if the contents of the exosomes could be engineered to contain signals, designed to be amplified and have a positive effect? It would be an extraordinary tool for regenerative medicine. Likewise, it would be exciting to farm some of the most biologically active molecules already present in our physiology.

This exosome frontier is exciting and is begging for more exploration. The key to the future of exosomes will be how well we explore it, how little we stumble in the process, and how we deliver it to patients. Currently, without a rigorous analysis of secreted molecules, without an understanding of what the secreted molecules do, and without strict parameters that create repeatable "crops," we have a long way to go.

In the meantime, there are more whole and balanced options for biologics, allografts, and regenerative medicine. Exosomes, depending on the stimulus and harvest protocols, also introduce the possibility of an unbalanced and unregulated overdose of "waste" molecules that can lead to teratogenesis or other unwanted adverse effects. This reaffirms the need for further understanding of all the aspects of exosome manufacture (see Appendix 3: Growth and Immune Regulating Factors, pages 63 and 64).

For now, the whole birth waste, not only exosomal content but the umbilical cord and placenta, offers a safer interim solution – even though *that* is also not fully understood.

ANIMAL STEM CELL PRODUCTS

Stem cell research and treatment did not start with human subjects. It started with animals, whose sacrifices led to medical developments and discoveries. The use of stem cells in veterinary medicine is irreplaceable and ever-evolving. Much of the knowledge we gained in the field of regenerative medicine, including stem cells, comes from animal research, utilizing veterinary facilities and animal laboratories. It is not wise to translate animal studies directly to humans, but they provide the building blocks of our medical knowledge.

In principle, stem cell use in animals parallels human use. Horses, cats, and dogs may benefit from stem cell treatment based on the same principles as their human friends. Treatment of the musculoskeletal system is the most common, but other applications have also been explored.[50] As in humans, both autologous and allogeneic stem cells are used. Bone marrow,[51] fat,[52][53] and blood-derived stem cell use is reported.[54][55] The key is not to implant stem cell material cross-species. Remember: umbilical cord stem cells from horses are good for horses, not for cats.

One of the major barriers to harvesting stem cells in animals is that umbilical cord stem cells are usually collected via c-section, which for obvious reasons, is not the normal delivery method for animals.

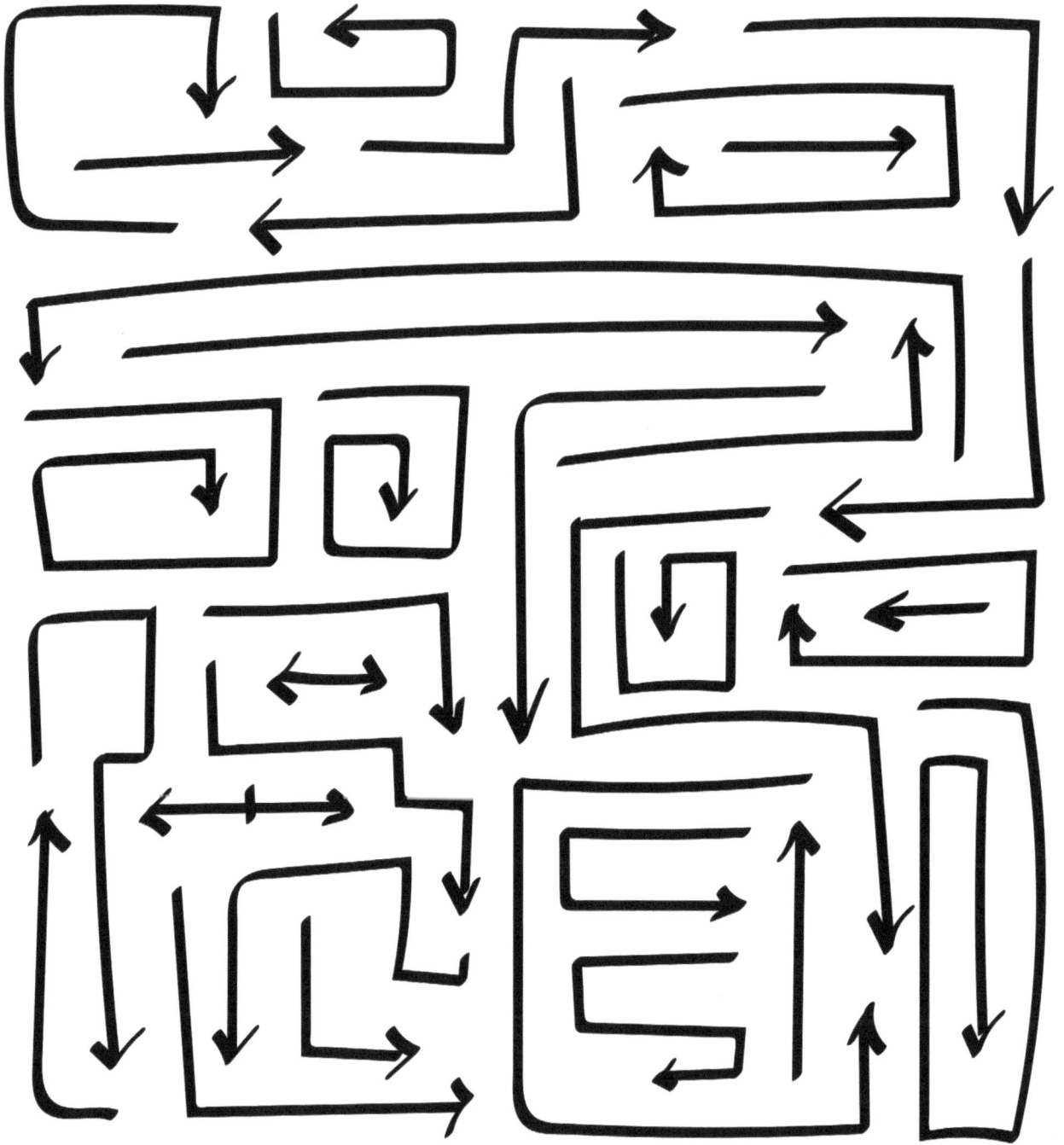

PART TWO:

PROBLEMS & CONCERNS

Many challenges must be overcome before stem cell treatment can be widely adopted. These include stem cell harvesting, concentrating, preserving, testing for diseases, increasing survivability, and so on. To gain the required knowhow will be expensive and time-consuming. But the reward is great: a novel therapeutic tool that may better countless lives.

Risks of stem cell treatment

Many patients, especially the devout, will approach stem cell treatment with a false preconception about how stem cells are harvested. This is a basic complication that can be averted through education: *Embryos are not used to harvest stem cells in the United States.* The same cannot be said for other countries.

Clinically, as with any treatment, there are other possible complications that must always be carefully considered. The stem cell DNA may mutate in the lab while the sample is processed. There may be an immune reaction within a sample or a disease transmission. Once cells are administered, they may experience aberrant differentiation, which can cause tumors. Finally, at the time of writing, most stem cell treatments are expensive and of unproven efficacy.[56][57]

Religious concerns

Stem cell therapy has been viewed negatively by those who feel it is immoral and against God's will. Many do not understand the stem cells used for therapy come from either excess birth material or the patients themselves. *Stem cells used for human treatment in the United States DO NOT come from fetuses or embryos.*

The big question is whether humans were meant to harness the miraculous ability of stem cells to treat pain, wounds, and other medical conditions. Ask yourself how God works. Do miracles suddenly appear from thin air? Or might we see God's hand in the miracles, large and small, produced by scientists, doctors, engineers, even random strangers? Cutting-edge research, out-of-the-box theories, viewing life's elements from a different angle are all random acts of kindness that have effectively led to miracles for countless people.

In today's world of medicine, stem cell therapy is both a biological miracle and an act of kindness to those suffering from ailments that are not easily treated. Miracles are a choice. They tend to take effort. The doctors, scientists, and other contributors to the development of stem cell therapy have done so to help those who are suffering. Their efforts have paid off with what seems to be an effective treatment. It would be immoral to refuse this therapy for patients.

EMBRYONIC STEM CELLS

At the dawn of stem cell research, some allogeneic stem cells were derived from aborted embryos. These **embryonic stem cells** (ESCs) were the source of serious moral, ethical, and religious concerns. Clinically, embryonic stem cells also proved unreliable. Outcomes were plagued with complications. Due to the complexities in their genetic composition and state of development, transplanted embryonic cells homed into the wrong areas and often suffered from uncertain differentiation, maturing into unwanted tissue, including cancer.

The use of animal-derived stem cells was also clinically problematic due to the dangers of cross-species tissue transplantation. These uncertainties and unknowns led to regulatory concerns and a change in public opinion, which lead to a drastic reduction in the clinical use of stem cells in Europe.

Due to media sensationalism, many still associate present-day stem cell treatment with ESCs. To repeat: *No human or animal ESCs are permitted for clinical use in the United States.*

UMBILICAL CORD STEM CELLS

In the United States, vendors of umbilical cord products collect stem cells from the donated birth waste of healthy live newborns delivered by C-section to avoid contamination. We already know that, by definition, embryonic stem cells, originate from developing fetal tissue. Umbilical cord-derived stem cells (UCSCs), on the other hand, are undifferentiated (meaning undeveloped) stem cells. UCSCs to date have *not* been associated with oncogenesis (do not cause healthy cells to turn into cancer cells) nor do they themselves turn into cancer.

Furthermore, harvesting from the umbilical cord sidesteps the ethical and religious concerns associated with embryonic stem cells. The improved clinical outcomes, coupled with their lack of moral hazards, have made umbilical cord stem cells popular for research and clinical applications. Nonetheless, a great deal more study of the potential use of UCSCs is necessary. Present-day clinical use is entirely investigational.

OVERSEAS STEM CELL TREATMENT

Many Americans travel abroad for stem cell treatment, trusting in fantastical claims about what can optimistically be described as questionable stem cell products. You will never quite know what you are getting. Overseas, stem cells may be manipulated and grown in a medium, a process that may influence their identity (phenotype) such that they are no longer stem cells, but fibroblasts, for instance. As a result, out of a claimed 100 million cells, only a few thousand may actually be stem cells (see also "Donor and tissue screening," page 35).

Better treatment and better products are available in the US, where stem cells are heavily regulated for the sake of public safety. Just about everything, from harvesting and testing to preservation and distribution, is under scrutiny. This is for the safety of the donors, patients, and the stem cells. Laboratory and physician accountability in this country is higher than just about anywhere else. Also, restrictions on animal and embryonic stem cells relieve ethical concerns about stem cell research and treatments.

The US prohibition on stem cell manipulation, expansion (growing in a lab), and enhancement add another level of protection. Stem cell expansion outside of the body, an unregulated practice at many overseas stem cell tourism destinations, increases the risk of tumorigenesis. That bears repeating: *Many stem cell tourism destinations do not regulate stem cell manipulation, which poses a higher cancer and contamination risk for patients.* The danger of stem cell expansion and enhancement is just one more reason to seek the most naive and least expanded product possible to administer to patients.[58]

Future research will undoubtedly bring more knowledge for safe and beneficial stem cell expansion and manipulation. We are not there yet.

The cost of care, as well, remains an issue. Stem cell treatment is expensive due to the sophisticated process of bringing fragile live material to a patient. Repeated treatments are also usually required, especially for complex conditions. The prospect of a single stem cell treatment curing a chronic illness is not realistic. Any travel abroad for such miraculous treatment would likely end in disappointment. Nevertheless, safer and more affordable alternatives are available for patients seeking treatment in the United States.

REGULATION

Responsible FDA-regulated vendors of umbilical cord products collect their biomaterials directly from the donated birth waste of healthy live newborns, making these products both ethical and practical.

Stem cell research was never banned in the US, but restrictions on funding were put in place during the George W. Bush administration. The stance was softened when President Bush signed into law the Stem Cell Therapeutic and Research Act of 2005, which provided $265 million for adult stem cell therapy, umbilical cord blood, and bone marrow treatment, and authorized $79 million for the collection of cord blood. In 2009, President Obama lifted restrictions on federal funding for stem cell research.

Bone marrow-derived stem cells have been used for decades to treat leukemia and lymphoma. This treatment is a covered benefit under some insurance policies. A number of hematopoietic stem-cell products derived from umbilical cord blood are currently approved by the FDA for the treatment of blood and immunological diseases.[59] However, for the majority of health conditions, stem cell treatments remain experimental and investigational – but not illegal.

Several laboratories offer stem cells to medical providers. Thanks to the growing availability and reliability of supply, stem cells have become part of the clinical arsenal. Stem cell treatment, when incorporated in an overall patient care plan, potentially opens new horizons in medicine, allowing for more effective treatments. Nevertheless, none of these applications are without limitations.

Biological products such as stem cells are defined in title 21 of the code of federal regulations, section 1271. Also, companies that produce, clean, test, and distribute stem cells have to adhere to multiple protocols established by specialty companies, tissue banks, blood blanks, the FDA, and the Center for Biological Evaluation and Research.[60]

The marketing of biologic therapies is also regulated. As an example, in May 2019, the Food and Drug Administration (FDA) warned a Scottsdale, Arizona company that it may be subject to prosecution for marketing unapproved stem cell products to treat a variety of diseases and conditions. Acting FDA Commissioner Ned Sharpless said: "We continue to see companies and individuals use questionable marketing campaigns to take advantage of vulnerable patients and their families with unproven claims about their unapproved stem cell products." [61]

WHAT IS PROHIBITED?

As mentioned earlier, cross-species animal stem cell treatment is not recommended, and human embryonic stem cells are not permitted for clinical use.

At the time of writing, the FDA does not allow any modification of stem cells, such as outside-the-body expansion (multiplying stem cells in a laboratory) or sorting (separating different cells on the basis of some parameter). The idea of making stem cells somehow better through scientific manipulation holds promise and likely will become a clinical reality in the future. But for now, as already mentioned, this is only performed in a laboratory setting, primarily overseas.

Recently a California lab was closed for mixing stem cells with viruses and injecting this mixture into patients' cancerous tumors. The idea of having stem cells activating viruses and working together makes sense. However, such stem cell use is not allowed in clinical practice currently due to unacceptable risk and lack of safety data. Currently, no manipulation of stem cells is permitted. However, there are clinical trials where a certain class of stem cells has been selected for use, such as with several Mesoblast trials (www. mesoblast.com).

With sufficient research, manipulation of stem cells may be more accepted and even surpass unaltered stem cell efficacy. The time for this practice has yet to come.

Donating stem cells

There are many social questions surrounding stem cell donations. Some have answers, and others do not. Federal guidelines outline what happens when a mother wants to preserve her newborn's umbilical cord stem cells. These guidelines regulate the collection, processing, testing, banking, packaging, and distribution of stem cells.[62]

Suppose new parents do collect and preserve a newborn's umbilical cord stem cells at birth. Can parents or another relative use the baby's preserved cells? The FDA allows the use of stem cells in first and second-degree relatives,[63] but this practice is ethically questionable. The sample ought to be reserved for the baby from which it was derived. If not, one can envision bad-actor scenarios in which desperate parents have more children simply for the purpose of providing stem cells for another "sick" child – or for themselves. What if relatives use up the entire sample before the child grows up? What if the child, late in life, discovers a need for his or her cells?

The use of an anonymous allogeneic umbilical cord-derived stem cell product avoids these ethical quandaries. It also addresses the problem of cell vitality after decades-long preservation. An anonymous sample might also be more financially attractive for the patient, as it would not come with the price tag of lifelong storage.

Donor and tissue screening

Donating umbilical cord tissue is voluntary and free. The mother has to be mentally capable of making decisions. Family screening, viral, bacterial, and immunologic screenings are all done. In a clinical setting, the cells cannot be modified, induced, expanded, enhanced, or altered in any way. Animal medium (including bovine serum) cannot be legally used in the US to multiply cells outside of the mother's body.

The testing is automated and allows for analyzing the content of growth factors, cytokines, mutations, RNA, DNA, and proportion of live and dead cells. Depending on the donor, umbilical cord blood contains anywhere from hundreds of thousands to millions of stem cells. Wharton's jelly contains even more cells, but it would be a mistake to think that all those cells are stem cells or mesenchymal stem cells for that matter.

Counting stem cells in a blood/tissue sample is a daunting process. The difference between cell types is not obvious, and they cannot be easily identified. This is why the number of stem cells in a sample is only a rough approximation. One would be wise to turn a skeptical eye on any company's

Examples of Donor Screening
Competency screening
Parental social screening
Viral and bacterial infectious disease screening
Genetic screening
Tryptic Soy Agar sterility test on both mother and cord blood to test for diseases and abnormalities

claims on a cell count for their product. A reputable vendor should perform appropriate cell selection such as FACS/cell sorting with appropriate markers and control.

Examples of Umbilical Cord Tissue Testing
Cytomegalovirus IgG and IgM
West Nile Virus Nucleic Acid Test
Zika Virus PCR test and IgM
Human T-lymphotropic virus I and II antibodies
HIV Type I and II and O antibodies
RPR (nontreponemal)
CAPITA (treponemal)
Hep. B antibody, antigen, and nucleic acid test
Hep. C antibodies and Nucleic Acid Test

Recently a new technology was developed by collaborative research at the Universities of Maryland, Pennsylvania, and Emory University. A process called "liquid biopsy" monitors transplanted stem cells by analyses of exosomes that are secreted by transplanted stem cells. Various proteins, nucleic acids, and micro ribonucleic acids are sorted to determine whether stem cell therapy will be effective for an individual patient, according to Dr. Kaushal of the University of Maryland. It was found that the contents of the exosomes in live organisms differed substantially from what they had produced in the lab, indicating the cells changed after transplantation.[64] This process still does not determine how many cells were transplanted but allows for an estimate of their clinical efficacy.

VITALITY AND PRESERVATION

Like all cells, stem cells require an adequate environment to survive. Outside the body, they die easily. Crowding, pressure, needle gauge, freezing, thawing, and chemical influences (like lidocaine, for instance) are just a few things that are potentially dangerous to stem cells.

Stem cells are at their best when freshly processed. Ideally, they should be used even before the sample is frozen, which requires proximity between the lab and the treatment center.[65][66][67]

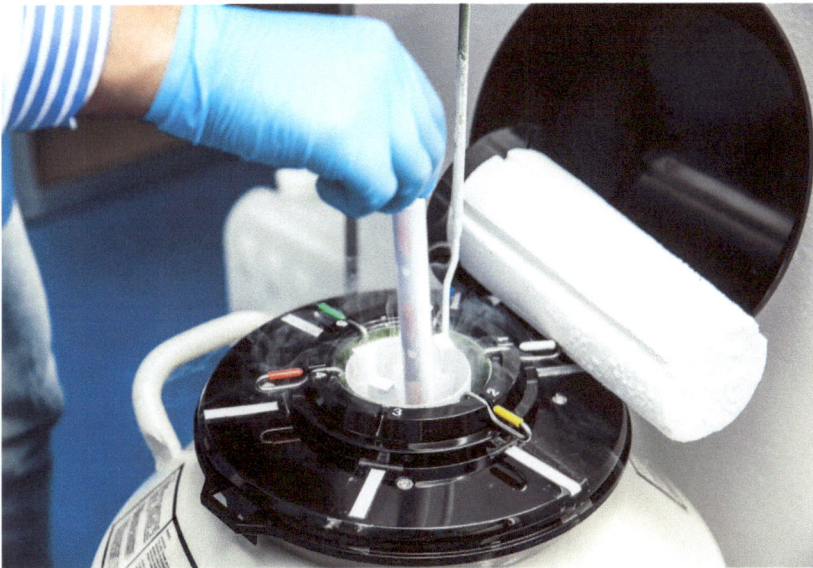

Liquid nitrogen cryotank used to preserve stem cells.

Although adult stem cell use is prevalent clinically, it represents older technology. However, autologous adult stem cells offer some advantages. For one, there is no need for preservatives. The cells are harvested, then promptly administered. Second, the risk of rejection is very low unless mutation or contamination occurs between the harvest and graft. However, this treatment is more expensive than PRP because of the collection process. Up to 40% of bone marrow-derived stem cells are hematopoietic and, therefore, likely of suboptimal efficacy for the repair of tissues such as muscles, tendons, and ligaments.

Imperfect harvesting and preservation, including storage at too high a temperature, may be detrimental to stem cell survival. Liquid nitrogen is the standard medium used for cryopreservation, but short-term shipment may be made on dry ice.

Dimethyl sulfoxide (DMSO), a standard preservative, is considered safe by the FDA but is known to be associated with liver and kidney damage. Many laboratories disclose that minimal concentrations of this chemical do not harm stem cells. Other companies make a point of not using it on the grounds that DMSO is cytotoxic in higher concentrations.[68] Though DMSO holds cells stable against cryopreservation (freezing), it may damage preserved cells over the long term.

Nevertheless, per Holm F. et al., contemporary cell freezing techniques offer very good cellular survival without much in the way of deleterious effects upon subsequent proliferation, as serum and xeno-free chemically-defined freezing procedures provide over 90% cell viability upon thawing.[69]

Glycerol is another accepted preservative. The major benefit of glycerol as a preservative is the increase in stability and survivability of the stem cells as well as a reduction of possible systemic reaction in comparison to DMSO products. This allows for the plausibility of giving higher stem cell dose with a lesser risk of adverse effects. Glycerol does make the stem cell sample more viscous, which can present a technical problem when injecting the cells.

GRAFT-VERSUS-HOST DISEASE

Graft-versus-host disease is probably the biggest concern for any practitioner who deals with foreign matter transplants into the human body. Even your own autologous stem cells can be rejected by your own body if they have DNA mutations, or are influenced by toxins, radiation, or nutritional stress. Umbilical cord stem cells, unlike adult stem cells, are immune naive. Lacking immune expression, they are less likely to provoke a response by the recipient's immune system (see "Autologous and allogeneic stem cells," page 15). In fact, umbilical cord stem cells are shown to minimize the active rejection process by repairing inflammation and optimizing the immune system. With time, this property may find an application in post-transplant treatment to improve tissue regeneration and reduce reliance on immunosuppressants when recovering from organ transplants.[70][71][72] Much needs to be done to research and prove the safety of this concept.

PART THREE:

CLINICAL APPLICATION

Although the clinical use of stem cells remains strictly investigational, stem cell treatments are slowly being introduced. The most widespread application is for connective tissue treatments – sports injuries, joint issues, muscle healing, and the like. This field of medicine has helped establish safety protocols and best practices for delivering stem cell treatment.

Stem cell outcome language is still developing. Do stem cells cure? Do they repair, restore, recover, improve? It seems all those words may be used, and all the clinical outcomes are possible, including an ambitious redefinition of "cure."[73][74][75]

My own clinic has hands-on experience with many conditions, mostly associated with pain. Though the anecdotal experience of clinicians and patients described below is relevant and revealing, many more studies must be undertaken to collect and prove the facts before scientifically-based clinical recommendations can be issued. Specific applications of stem cells in clinical practice are not FDA-approved. They remain experimental and investigational. Many specific methods of administration are also not yet approved.

PATIENT EXPERIENCE

Most patients would say their trips to the doctor are boring. Stem cells tend to make appointments more interesting. If the patient receives a stem cell infusion via IV, it starts like any other infusion: a stick in a vein to start an IV. It may not be the most pleasant experience, but it is usually no big deal.

Then comes the exciting part: a frozen vial filled with stem cells. We usually ask the patient to help thaw the vial in the palm of their hand. This may be a good psychological way to "bond" with stem cells, so to speak. Thawing can also be done in body temperature water or by sitting at room temperature until the vial is completely thawed.

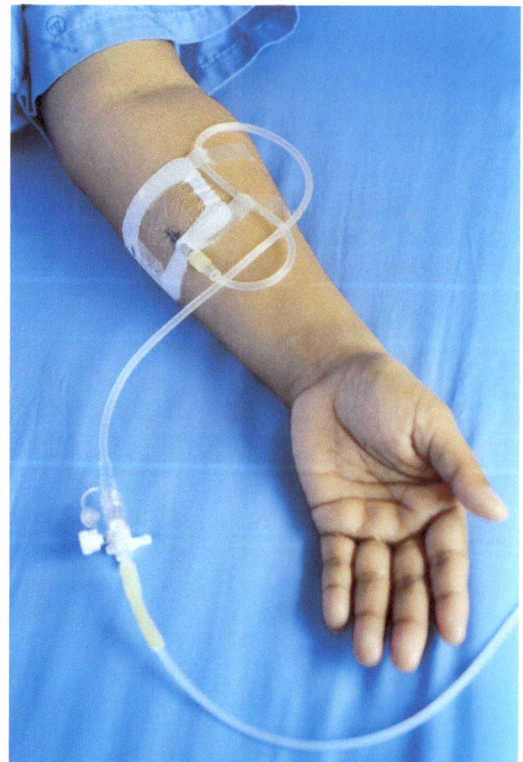

A stem cell intravenous infusion looks and feels no different than any other infusion.

Every vial has an associated tracking number that allows the supplier to trace it back to the source (the donor), should the need for investigation arise. A larger bore needle is used for easier flow and is less traumatic for the stem cells. The cells are introduced into the IV tubing through a slow push from a syringe with normal saline to assure that almost all of the cells make it to the patient. Some clinics infuse vitamins and nutrients alongside stem cells. Myer's cocktail – a recipe that varies but usually consists of magnesium, calcium, vitamins B and C – is popular but tends to be done for psychological reasons rather than any proven efficacy.

Immediate adverse effects are uncommon and are normally associated with the venipuncture rather than the stem cells. Some patients experience heaviness in their legs or in the whole body, which is difficult to explain but disappears quickly. A flu-like sensation lasting for a few days has been reported at times.

Stem cell injections in joints, muscles, and other areas of the body are no different from medication injections in those same areas. Stem cells cause initial local (and healthy!) inflammation; temporary swelling can be expected. A day or two of pain increase is also likely. Sometimes the pain may be very pronounced and requires a few doses of oral pain medication. Superficial analgesia with lidocaine may be carefully done, but mixing it with stem cells is contraindicated as lidocaine interferes with stem cell viability. The same goes for steroids. We recommend not using steroids for at least two weeks before and four weeks after stem cell treatment. This applies to both local and IV treatment. However, if the patient's condition does not allow for the discontinuation of steroids, stem cell treatment may still be conducted.

POST-TREATMENT GUIDELINES

In the majority of cases, post-stem cell treatment recommendations are simple: avoid strenuous activity, stay hydrated, and maintain a healthy diet. If problems occur, report them to your doctor as soon as possible.

When stem cells are injected into large joints, some additional care is needed. The transplanted stem cells need time before they can tolerate stress. There is limited published literature about the exact guidelines for physical therapy (PT) after stem cell treatments.

The general consensus is to avoid high-impact activities for about three months post-injection. The intensity of PT sessions should be reduced by about 25% during the first two weeks and increase slowly over the course of about eight weeks. If the patient lifts weights, decrease the weight by about 25-50%, depending on how heavy the weights were to start with (decrease moderate weights by 25% and heavy weights by 50%) and gradually increase over the course of eight to twelve weeks (see Appendix 4 for more information).

The question of acupuncture is also open. Acupuncture itself is unlikely to impede stem cells and actually may even enhance their function, but the use of electro-acupuncture is controversial. Until more is known, it is probably better to avoid electro-acupuncture, moxibustion, or cupping for at least two to three weeks post stem cell treatment.

DURATION OF STEM CELL ACTION

We do not know for sure how long transplanted stem cells live. It depends on the environment they are put in, the diseases the patient has, the kinds of medications the patient is on, and numerous other factors, most of which are unknown at this time.

The duration of stem cell action depends on the age at harvesting and the transplant niche. Neural tissue, soft tissue, cartilage, and bone all have very different local conditions that can significantly limit the possible beneficial effects. Concentrated adult stem cells do have therapeutic potential, just not as much as young stem cells (see "Telomeres and aging," page 21).

WHAT ABOUT MULTIPLE CONDITIONS?

It stands to reason that a patient with 25 diseases would be unlikely to respond to stem cell treatment as well as someone with a single disease (see "What happens to stem cells in the body?" page 10). Severe diseases will not respond as well as milder conditions. The number of treatments and dosage depends on such factors. The older you are, the more difficult it is to repair tissues. Younger people are expected to improve faster, and the results may last longer. The health of the immune and endocrine systems may aid or impair treatment response.

My patients frequently express surprise that the condition they wanted to treat did not improve as much as some other ailment in their body. We presently cannot direct cells to target a particular problem. Stem cells select their battles for themselves, especially in intravenous administration. A sufficient number of treatments may provide enough cells to attend to most conditions. But stem cells should not be viewed as a cure-all. Repeated treatments are frequently needed, and it is unwise to expect guaranteed recovery.

STEM CELLS AND MEDICATIONS

It is known that lidocaine is toxic to stem cells as it is to many other cells, including cartilage, which complicates tissue injections. Steroids also are not safe in combination with stem cells.

Cancer treatment medications are designed to kill rapidly-dividing cells and, consequently, are likely to impair or kill stem cells. Any stem cell treatment on cancer patients, if undertaken at all, should be done between cycles or after the course of chemotherapy.

INTRAVENOUS ADMINISTRATION

Generalized conditions, especially auto-immune diseases such as rheumatoid arthritis, myasthenia gravis, lupus, Crohn's disease, interstitial cystitis (IC), and others cannot be successfully treated with local injections.[76][77][78][79] Utilization of stem cells, especially blood-derived, also makes sense in uncontrollable infections or hard-to-treat conditions such as Lyme disease. Stem cells are furthermore shown to increase egg count and sperm vitality, which suggests their use in infertility problems. [80][81] However, the intravenous route of administration is more controversial and less researched than many other applications. If infused intravenously, stem cells are carried to the lungs, where they settle and multiply for about two weeks. After this time, they leave the lungs and distribute themselves to the areas of need.[82][83][84] This activity has yet to be proven and likely depends on many factors, known and unknown. It is likely that other organs such as the gut and spleen may filter stem cells and diminish the numbers that arrive at the target site. The thymus is also involved in attracting stem cells.

There is a remarkable mystery in the mechanism of stem cell-associated improvement. The treatment does not so much "fix" immune conditions as it modulates them, just as a leg prosthesis allows an amputee to walk. Our patients frequently show objective improvement in their auto-immune symptoms without the consequent improvement in laboratory markers. The same applies to lung conditions: When a person stops using oxygen, blood oxygen levels normalize while objective lung tests may remain abnormal. However, the placebo effect cannot explain the sustained improvement in Myasthenia Gravis or the increase in blood oxygen.

Prophylactic stem cell use, especially in IV formulation, is controversial. It may aid in longevity and illness prevention, though this is highly speculative at this time.

EPIDURAL INJECTIONS

Epidural injections may be considered for spinal root impingement, sciatica, bulging discs, and disc tear repair to replace epidural steroid injections. This is done in clinical practice but is highly experimental and not yet proven.

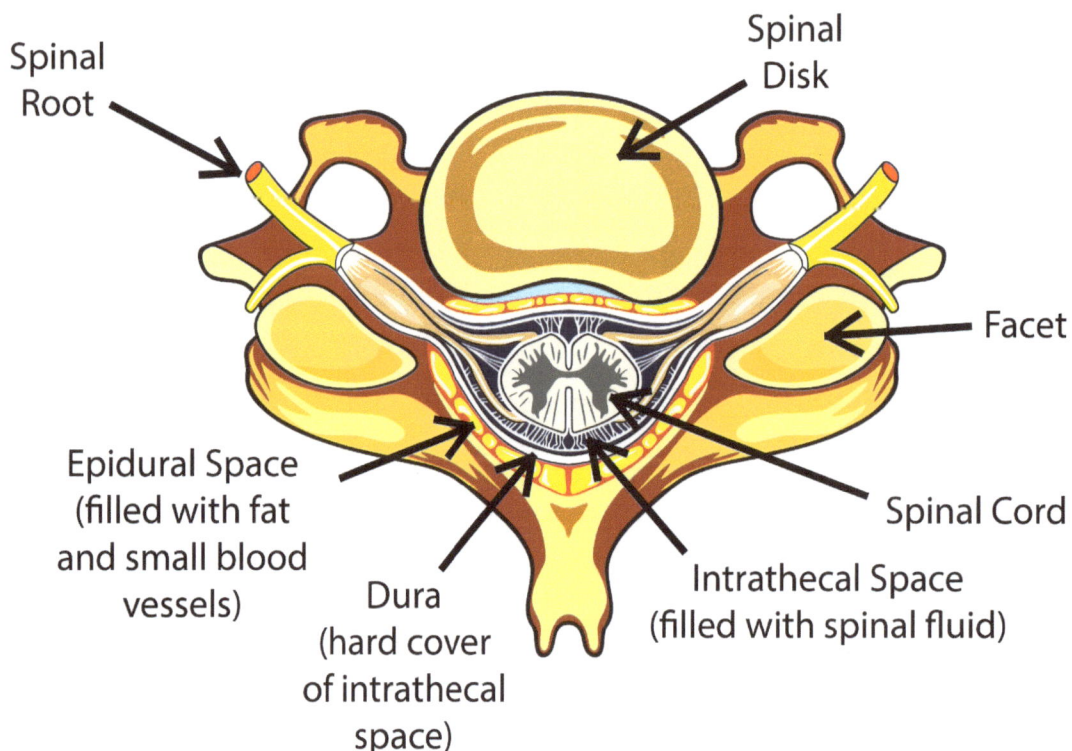

The spinal cord is protected by bones and cushioned by cerebrospinal fluid.

INTRATHECAL STEM CELL INTRODUCTION

Intrathecal stem cell introduction may be of value due to a theoretically higher penetration into the brain. Cerebrospinal fluid does not float like a river, carrying cells inside the brain. Rather it oscillates up and down. But due to a high concentration in the confined space, intrathecal stem cell introduction could possibly help with central nervous system diseases such as Parkinson's, Alzheimer's, ALS, Multiple Sclerosis, traumatic brain injury, spinal cord injury, and transverse myelitis.[85][86] As with all stem cell treatments, this remains experimental.

INTRA-ARTICULAR ADMINISTRATION

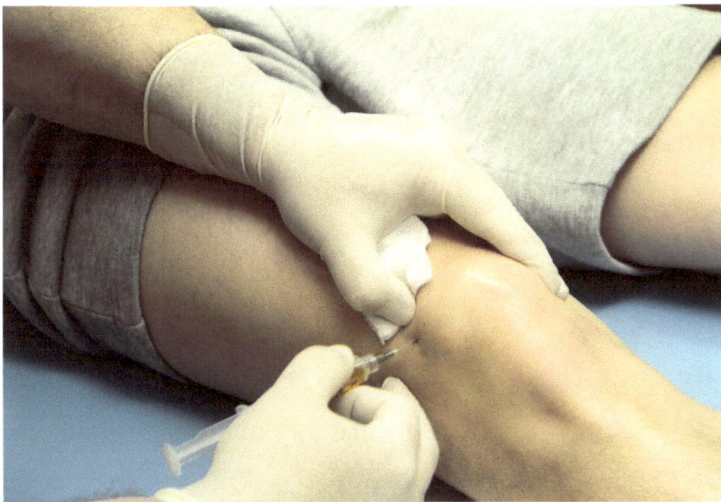

Ideally, knee joint injections are done under fluoroscopic (X-ray) guidance.

The oldest method of stem cell administration is intra-articular (IA/inside the joint). Like with PRP, stem cells are used to treat degenerative joint disease, labrum tears, spine facets, and sacroiliac joints. Clinically, stem cells may be injected right into the area of trouble with hope for repair.[87][88] Some insurance plans (mostly self-insured employer plans) have started to allow coverage of IA stem cell treatments, especially in the lower extremities and knees.

There is conflicting evidence about what happens to stem cells upon intra-articular injection in terms of survivability or destination. There is also conflicting evidence as to whether stem cells have a regenerative effect on cartilage. A few studies suggest that there may be some effect. One meta-analysis found no difference in MRI or range of motion in stem cell-injected osteoarthritic knees. At the same time, it did find suppression in pain, suggestive of the anti-inflammatory action of stem cell-secreted molecules.[89]

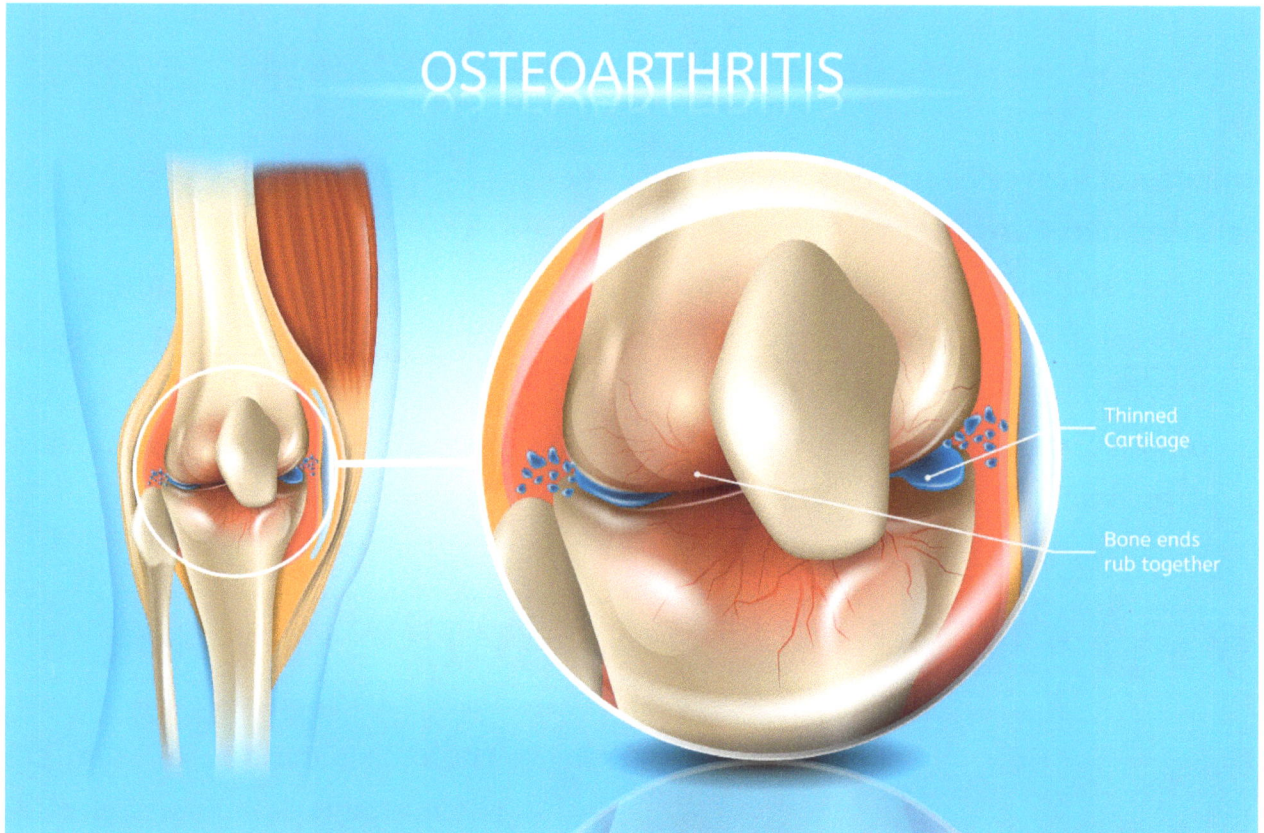

In knees affected by osteoarthritis, the cartilage thins/hardens, fragments break off, bones may develop microfractures; all causing pain. Bringing stem cells into this environment may assist healing and regeneration.

Just like the patients who, despite abnormal labs, reported improved function of the lungs or immune system, patients who receive intra-articular stem cell treatment frequently report sustained joint improvement despite imaging that may still show insufficient cartilage in the joint. We regularly see patients who avoid scheduled joint replacement and show good mobility while their X-rays and MRIs remain suboptimal. Presently we can only speculate how that is possible.

Intradiscal injections

Intradiscal injections for the treatment of degenerative disc disease, disc tear, bulging, and herniated discs make sense due to the core function of stem cells. Theoretically, mesenchymal cells may be of more value than hematopoietic cells in this application.[90][91] The efficacy of stem cells for disc injury is not at all clear with many contradictory studies and little evidence for transplant survival and action of the transplanted cells.

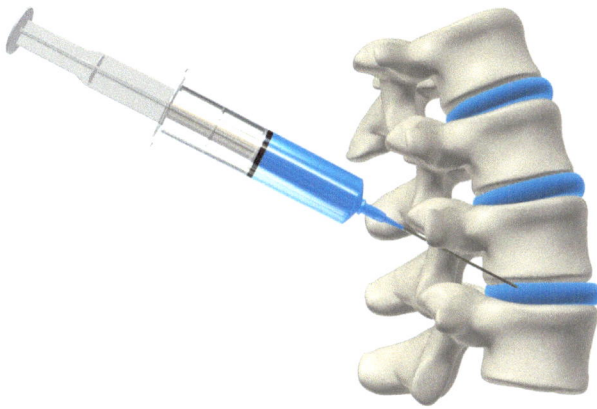

Illustration of an intradiscal injection.

The disc is a hypoxic, avascular, and ischemic (poor in oxygen) environment hostile to stem cells. Still, stem cells may assist in regeneration by the release of biologically active factors and improvement in vascularization and oxygenation of the surrounding tissues. There is a reason to consider injecting only some separated (or synthesized!) growth factors or whole "matrix" into a disk.

Stem cells may also be collected from a healthy nucleus pulposus (the soft inner part of the disc) and then injected into a diseased spinal disc. These precursor stem cells are further along the developmental pathway than umbilical cord stem cells. Nucleus pulposus stem cells that were differentiated in a lab setting demonstrated the remarkable but not unpredictable ability to become nerve cells. As such, they have the potential for neural repair in addition to connective tissue repair.[92]

In August 2019, the FDA granted Fast Track designation for an investigational cell therapy to reduce pain and disability associated with degenerative disc disease. This therapy uses a homologous, allogeneic, injectable cell therapy that utilizes patented progenitor cells, known as discogenic cells. The cells are derived from adult human intervertebral disc tissue and are injected into the target disc. This therapy may have an anti-inflammatory effect as well as the regenerative capacity to create new intervertebral disc tissue. The FDA is evaluating this product under an investigational new drug allowance and will be regulating it as a drug-biologic through a biologics license application.[93]

INTRAMUSCULAR INJECTIONS

Intramuscular introduction of stem cells is less controversial than other methods, though still experimental. This treatment was reported for a number of high-profile athletes. Autologous stem cells and PRP are also described as beneficial in this application. Nevertheless, the younger the stem cells, the better the potential outcome, so umbilical cord allogeneic cells may still be the choice over autologous adult cells.[94][95][96]

When injected into a large muscle, stem cells can travel some distance around the body. Although transplanted cells may migrate elsewhere, the majority will concentrate at the injection site to heal the injury.

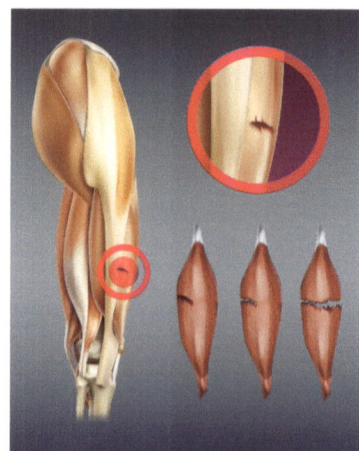

Ruptured muscles are hard to heal. Stem cells may help the process.

INTRALIGAMENT INJECTIONS

Intraligament injections may be considered for Achilles tendon repair, treatment of plantar fasciitis, and knee ligament restoration. Mesenchymal cells may be the right choice in this application.[97][98][99]

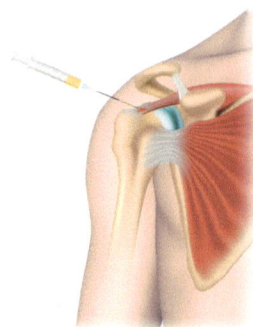

Shoulder injection.

TENDON RUPTURE

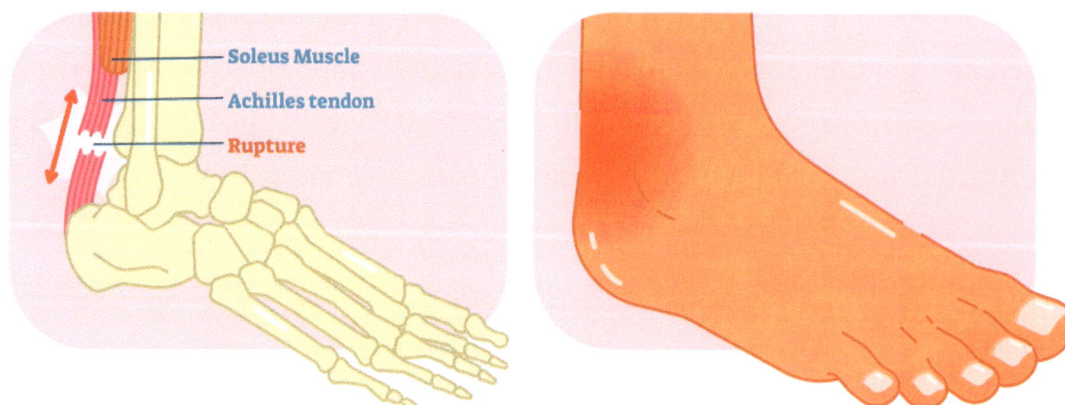

Soleus Muscle
Achilles tendon
Rupture

Injecting injured tendons with stem cells may accelerate healing. PRP is also effective for this treatment.

INTRAOSSEOUS INJECTIONS

Intraosseous (inside the bone) injections for the treatment of bone fractures and non-junction situations (when bones do not come together at the fracture site) are being explored. There is also a new study into parathyroid hormone aiding IV stem cells' ability to home to bone tissue for osteoporosis treatment. Fractures may heal faster; traumas and sports injuries may be amenable to stem cell treatment.[100 101 102]

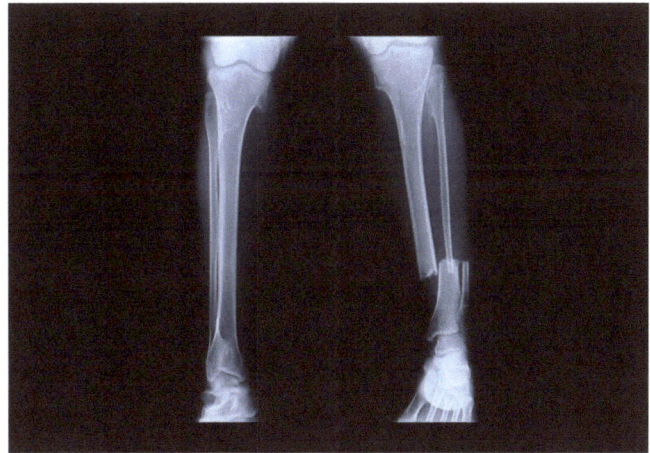

Proof that stem cells aid in bone healing, would revolutionize trauma treatment.

INTRACARDIAC INJECTIONS

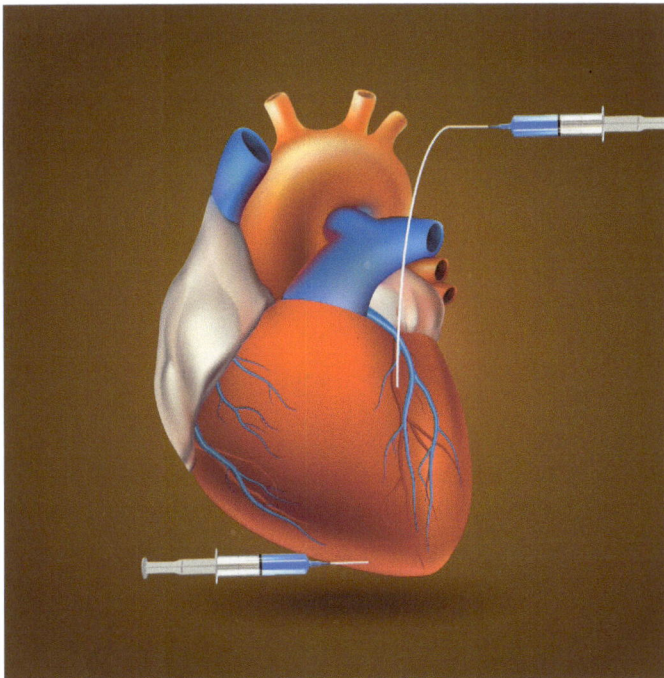

Introduction of stem cells into the heart.

Thanks to stem cell migration and homing inside the cardiac wall, cardiac repair after myocardial infarction may be achieved by intracardiac stem cell administration, cardiac artery stem cell infusion, or an IV treatment alike. Much research is going on in this area, but we still do not know enough to be certain of the outcomes of such treatments.[103 104 105 106]

In June 2019, the FDA granted Orphan Drug designation to a cell therapy that delivers allogeneic mesenchymal precursor cells in a single intra-myocardial injection. One day this may become a therapy to prevent post-implantation mucosal bleeding in end-stage chronic heart failure patients. This treatment is also investigated in a clinical trial involving patients with moderate to advanced heart failure.[107]

INTRAORGAN INJECTIONS

Similar in principle to intracardiac injection, other intraorgan stem cell administration is probably the least researched method, but will likely be of great service to future surgeons once the mechanism and efficacy of such treatments are established. One may envision the introduction of stem cells into the pancreas to battle diabetes, or into the liver, kidney, or other organs to treat corresponding diseases.

BRAIN AND INTRASPINAL TREATMENTS

During stem cell migration, some extracellular components may travel around the body and cross the blood-brain barrier, but much more research has to be done to claim this with certainty. However, stem cells are too big to penetrate into the brain if injected peripherally. The only way for stem cells to appear inside the central nervous system is by direct introduction.

Brain matter or intraventricular stem cell placement is far from routine clinical use. One day, stem cells may find their place in neurosurgery. The same applies to stem cell injections inside the spinal cord to treat severe cord injuries.[108] [109]

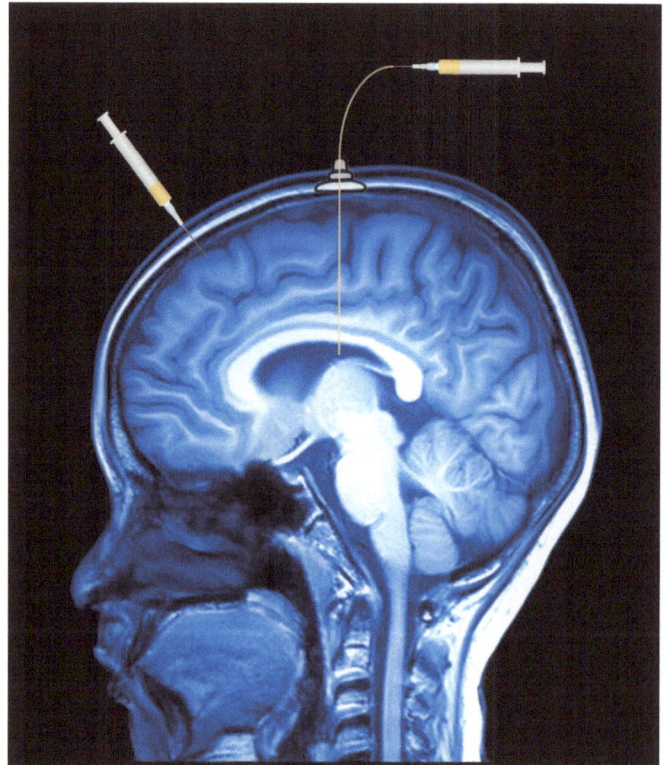

Infusion of stem cells inside ventricles or inside brain matter

At least four cases of spinal tumors have been reported following experimental nasal stem cell transplants for paralysis. It seems the risk of tumorigenesis increases when using an olfactory mucosal autograft, perhaps because the adult autologous cells contain more precursor than progenitor cells. This underlines the cancer risk of adult autologous cells.[110] Simply said, your own stem cells might not be as safe as you think.

Intraocular and eye surface treatment

Intraocular (inside the eye) injections may be disastrous and are not ready for human clinical use, though eye surface treatment is performed successfully by experienced ophthalmologists.[111] [112] [113] A clinic in Florida was closed after blinding several patients. The NIH sponsors ongoing studies of the appropriate use of stem cells in eye diseases.

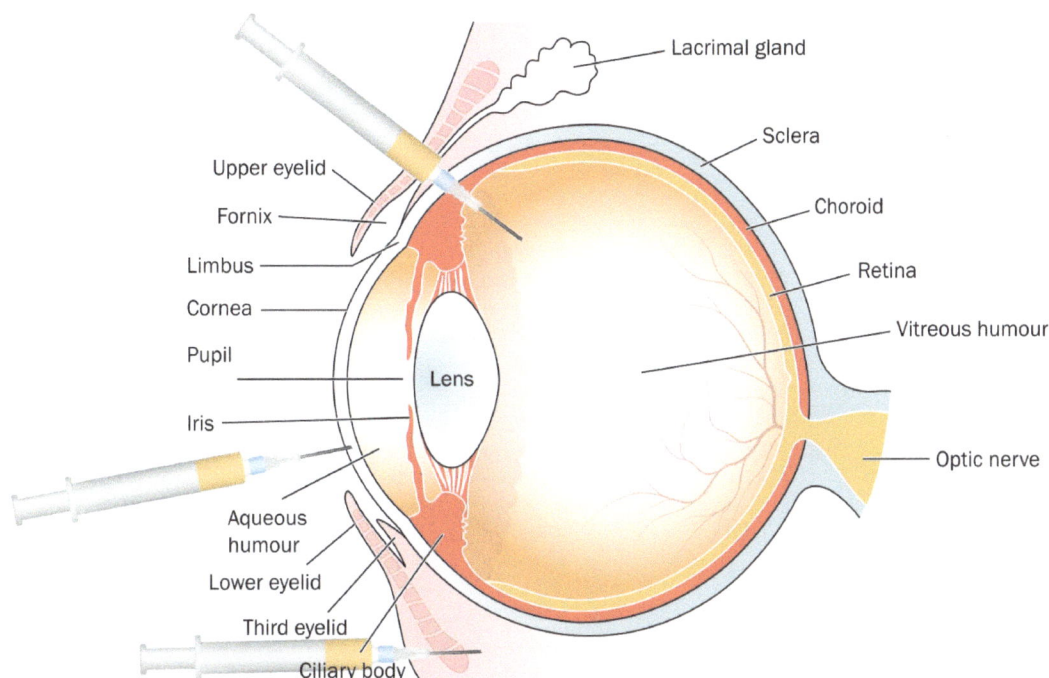

Stem cells may one day be placed in various eye compartments.
Much more research has to be done before clinical use is approved.

Stem cells and cancer

Treating cancer with stem cells is controversial. Although stem cells have been shown to treat multiple types of cancer, there is a danger of giving patients false hope. The use of costly experimental treatments for life-threatening diseases requires clear and informed patient consent.[114] [115] [116]

Stem cells may develop into cancerous tumors due to aberrant differentiation. Embryonic stem cells, which have been shown to turn into cancer cells, are considered especially risky from the standpoint of cancer treatment. There are also reports of adult stem cell involvement in tumorigenesis, as mentioned above.[117] [118] [119]

From what is known today, the cancer risk appears lowest with umbilical cord blood and Wharton's jelly stem cells, which so far have never been observed to develop into cancer (see "Amniotic and umbilical stem cell products," page 20).

Finally, because exosomes are a subset of the entire biologic milieu found in the umbilical cord, there is also a risk of tumorigenesis caused by the activating factors included within exosomes (see "Exosomes," page 25).[120][121] The risk heavily depends on the concentration and activity of exosomes that are introduced into the patient. This brings an important cautionary note: Too much stem cell treatment may be harmful. You can have "too much of a good thing." Since it is not presently known what is "too much" in relation to stem cells, caution against over-treatment should be the rule for both clinicians and patients.

CAN STEM CELLS BE USED TO TREAT PAIN?

There are a number of ways that stem cells may help pain. One is immediate, by blocking the initiation of the pain cascade and decreasing inflammation.[122][123] From clinical experience, pain also improves in a delayed fashion and is associated with tissue repair and oxygenation, improvement in metabolism, and boosting the immune system.[124][125][126]

DENTAL APPLICATIONS

Dental applications of stem cells are expanding, even to the point of growing new teeth. Local dental stem cell injections are logical in both tissue restoration and infection management.[127][128][129][130][131]

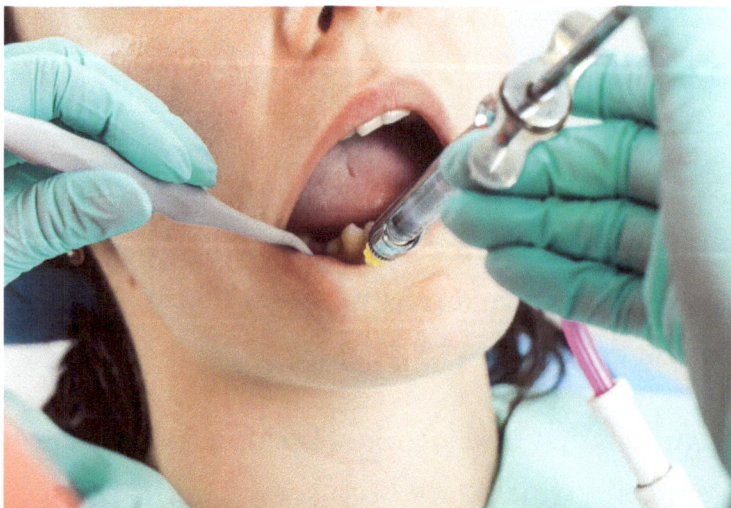

Dental stem cell injection

Cosmetic treatment

The cosmetic use of stem cells is intriguing. One day, there may be a place in medicine to grow and rejuvenate hair, skin, and fat pads.

A large enough needle bore has to be used, but scarring from large needle punctures, especially in the face, is of concern. Local anesthetics interfere with stem cell vitality, which complicates live stem cell injections in cosmetics. The extracellular component (matrix) does not require large-bore needles and may be administered through fine needles. Topical cosmetic stem cell use is fiction. Live stem cells cannot survive in a cream or an ointment. At the same time, the extracellular component or "serum," to borrow the term used in the cosmetic industry, may be of value if mixed with a chemical vehicle to take growth factors through the skin.[132][133][134]

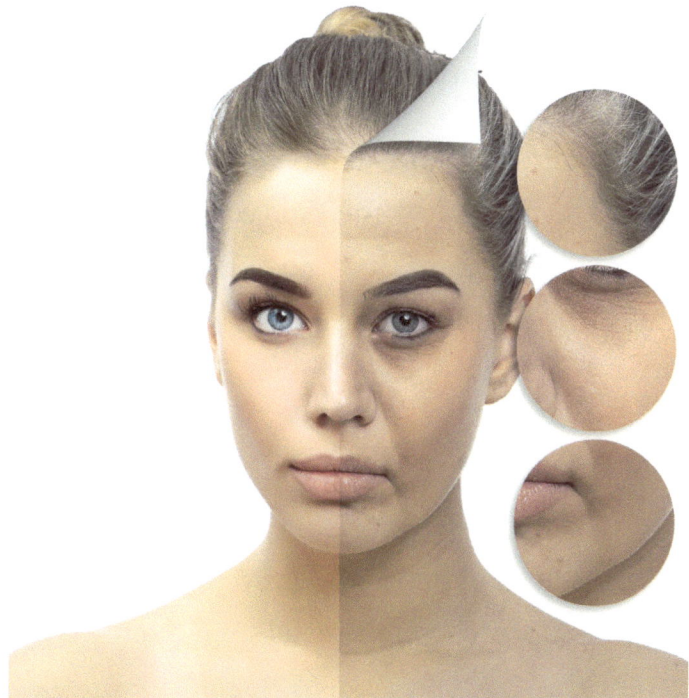

Skin, hair, and fat pad rejuvenation has been reported after stem cell treatments.

The most intriguing cosmetic possibility may be through intravenous infusion of stem cells. It is fanciful to contemplate that as stem cells continue to multiply and revitalize within the host – as new tissues replace older ones – stem cell treatments in a way make the recipient younger. To date, no human studies take aim at this possibility. It is unlikely that stem cells can reverse aging; but it is probable that the prophylactic use of umbilical cord stem cells, if started early enough, may slow aging and eventually make people appear younger than their calendar age. This has been shown to work in rats.[135] With so many unknowns concerning possible future complications of stem cell treatment, the choice of using umbilical stem cells prophylactically is a difficult one.

CAN STEM CELLS PROLONG LIFE?

A recent study published in the journal *Nature* showed that the aging process might be reversed when stem cells are introduced into a rat's brain, and the cells are then fooled into perceiving that their surroundings are soft and young.[136] The very fact that it is possible in rats does not mean that this would directly translate to humans, but the promise is there. We know for sure that stem cells are involved in slowing aging in many different ways.[137]

Other animal studies demonstrate a significant increase in longevity coupled with better health in the experimental subjects. If this effect translates to humans, we may have a better future that requires fewer doctors and hospitals.[138][139] This is a far-reaching statement, but isn't it the ultimate dream?

GROWING ORGANS

It seems to be impossible to grow missing organs without stem cell manipulation (presently illegal), so any current clinical stem cell use is confined to a repair of pre-existing damaged structures.

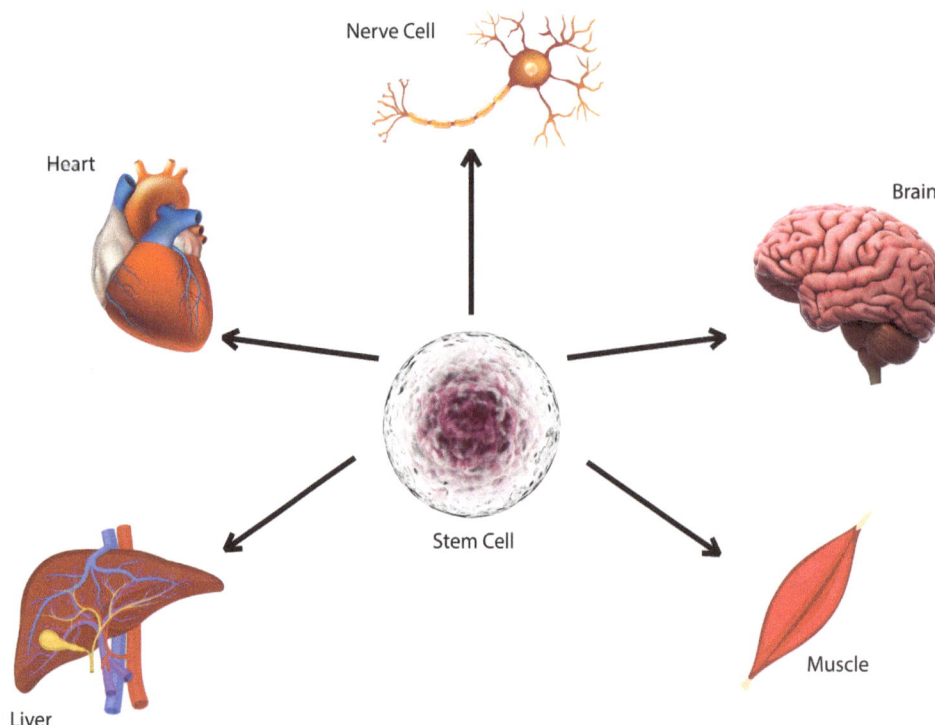

**Stem cells may become specialized tissue,
opening the door to rebuilding or even replacing damaged organs.**

SCAR FORMATION

Could stem cells be used to treat keloid scars or to prevent post-surgical scarring?[140] [141] [142] [143] Amniotic membrane seeded with stem cells can be used for the treatment of wounds and tissue defects. For example, a successful spina bifida tissue defect repair has been performed,[144] complete with newly-formed sweat glands, seborrheic glands, and hair follicles. The same kind of tissue repair has been seen in animal studies (earhole closure in mice).[145]

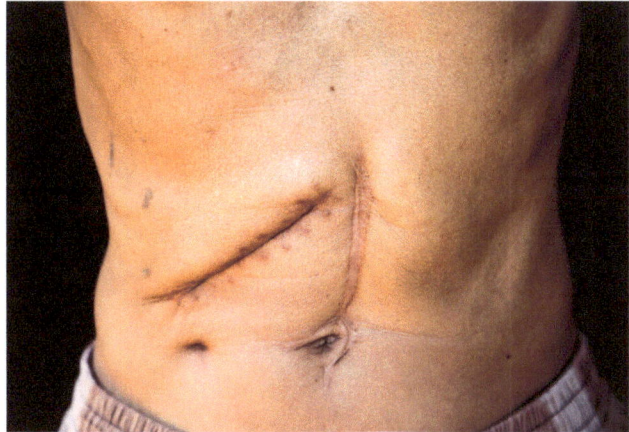

Treating and preventing skin and internal scar formation would help many patients.

MENTAL ILLNESS

As we know, multiple mental conditions are based on the inflammatory process. Psychosis, depression, autism, Alzheimer's dementia, traumatic brain injury, and many other diseases are inflammatory in nature. Theoretically, they can be treated with stem cells if it can be conclusively shown that stem cells do regulate inflammation. However, this remains speculative at present.[146] [147] [148] [149] [150] The use of stem cells has also been reported in the treatment of alcohol and stimulant addiction, but the clinical results are far from certain.[151] [152]

CONCLUSION

A new field of knowledge is always exciting. One feature is common in anything new and unexplored: difference in opinions. This is usually enriching and positive but is sometimes bitter and toxic. Extremists claim that only their opinion matters when, in fact, every approach is useful, depending on the circumstances. Applied to stem cells, this means that PRP, amniotic fluid, amniotic membrane, matrix, autologous, and allogeneic stem cells all have their place in medicine. We should be wary of those who claim that only one product or modality has any value.

So much about the whole world of stem cell treatment remains unknown. We still need to learn who to treat, what kind of stem cells products to use, and what indications stem cells may treat. The timing of stem cell treatment with respect to the patient's age and disease process remains unclear. The question of treatment boosters is still open. Should we wait until the patient's disease relapses, or should we repeat treatment before their disease gets worse? Combination treatment with medications is also unclear. Which medications aid or impair stem cells' efficacy and safety? What about electric, mechanical, or magnetic stimulation of tissues with stem cells? Do vitamins and nutrients affect stem cell function? If so, how? Years of research are needed to answer these and other questions. Hopefully, more research will help us maximize the safety and efficacy of stem cells in clinical practice.[153][154][155][156]

Innovation in medicine comes from both laboratory and clinical practice. Thousands of stem cell studies are underway around the world, half of them in the United States. Adult stem cells are being actively researched. Allogeneic stem cells, Wharton's jelly, and the cord blood are also studied (see Appendix 5: Current stem cell studies).

China recently issued draft regulations that would permit some hospitals to sell therapies, developed from patients' own cells, without approval from the nation's drug regulator. The International Society for Stem Cell Research (ISSCR) sent a statement outlining its concerns to China's National Medical Products Administration in Beijing, urging more research before the wide use of stem cells. This development points to a fragile balance of countervailing forces: innovation and regulation, efficacy and safety, medical and political – in short, risk and reward.

There is no easy match for the promise and pitfalls of stem cell research and treatment. The pharmaceutical model, which zeros in on a single molecule for exhaustive testing, does not apply to complex biological products such as stem cells. Governments do not know how to assure safety without suffocating fact-finding in stem cell research. A national registry is needed. Clinical outcomes need to be reported and analyzed. Stem cell laboratories need to be systematically reviewed and compared in a comprehensible and transparent manner. Patients need to be able to find appropriate treatment. Doctors and the public need to be educated. All this requires deep reservoirs of scientific brainpower, organizational genius, and institutional and political goodwill – as well as sufficient funding.

And yet the endeavor is worth the expense. We are constantly enriched by new knowledge. The clinical use of stem cells opens new horizons. At this time, stem cell treatment is reserved for otherwise untreatable conditions, but as our knowledge base and experience expands, we will likely witness a healthcare revolution.

Stem cell science develops quickly, and what seems to be true today may not be true tomorrow. This is the nature of any scientific field, and that is what makes learning a lifelong project. This book reflects what is known at the time of writing. I hope it will be a stepping stone for those who continue to be interested in stem cells.

A
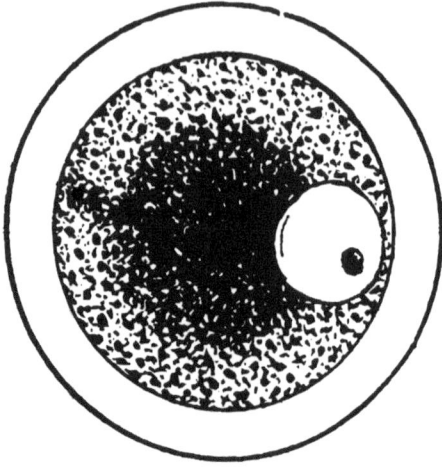

B
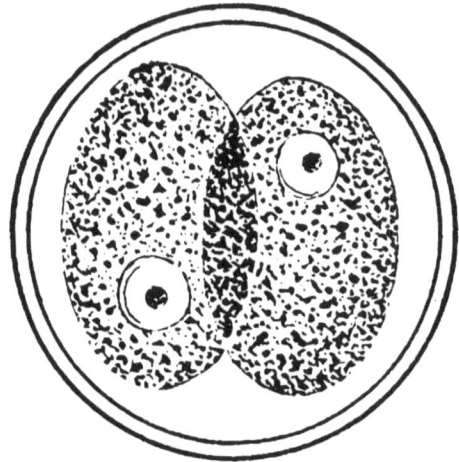

C
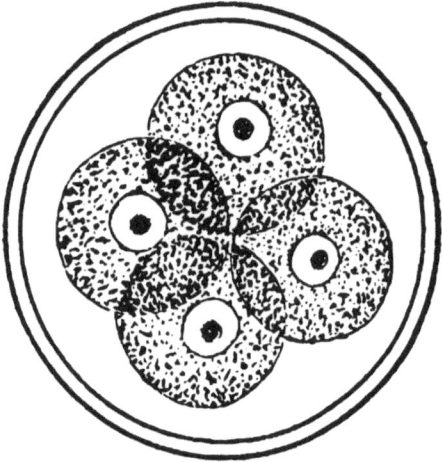

D
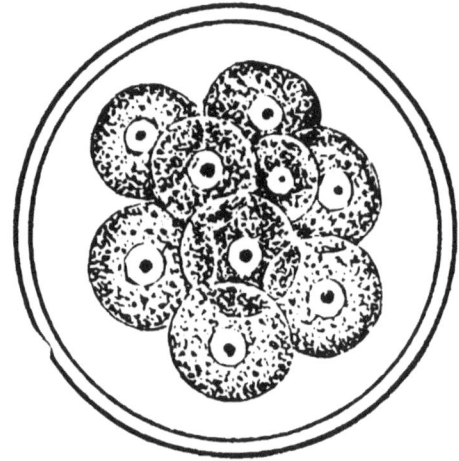

E
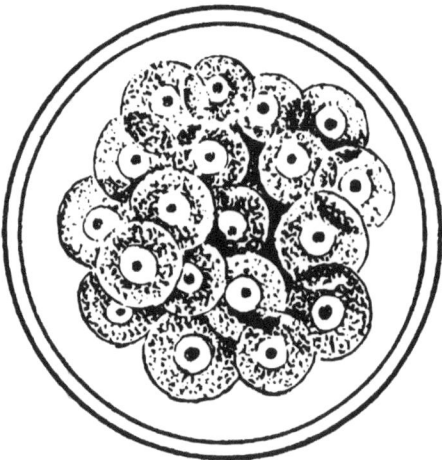

F
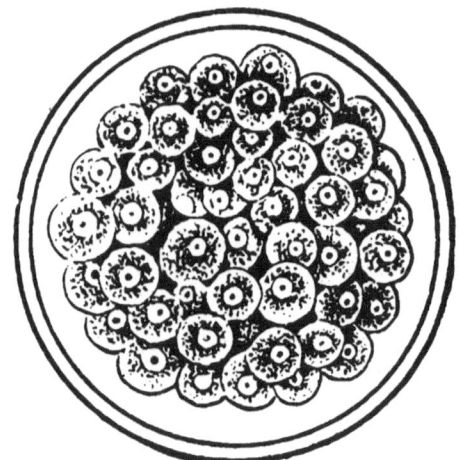

Vintage cell drawing

PART FOUR:

END MATTER

Appendix 1: Stem cell glossary

Term	Definition
allogeneic stem cells	stem cells from a donor other than the recipient
amniotic fluid	the liquid that cushions a growing fetus; it lacks live stem cells but is rich with cytokines and growth factors produced by stem cells
amniotic membrane	the lining of the embryonic sack; it is covered with stem cells and may be used topically as a healing barrier treatment for burns, wounds, etc.
animal stem cells	any animal tissue-derived stem cells
autologous stem cells	the patient's own stem cells used on him or herself
embryonic stem cells	stem cells derived from aborted embryos; the source of serious moral, ethical, and religious concerns; today no Embryonic Stem Cells are permitted for clinical use in the United States
exosomes	cellular sub-compartments of living cells; packaged with payloads of growth factors, cytokines, & other factors designed to secrete from the cells
hematopoietic stem cells	stem cells that are present primarily in blood and bone marrow; they differentiate into white and red blood cells and plasma components which aid the immune system; lymphocytes, monocytes, and macrophages also come out of this cell line, aiding in anti-inflammatory processes in the body
matrix	matrix lacks a precise definition and usually refers to an assembly of cytokines and growth factors derived from stem cells with no actual live stem cells in the composition
mesenchymal stem cells	these stem cells may come from anywhere in the body, but are especially prevalent in the umbilical cord wall; these stem cells mostly differentiate into connective tissue and are involved in organ repair
precursor stem cells	stem cells than can become a cell or a tissue of a particular type (i.e., ligaments, muscles or cartilage, and not endocrine cells)
progenitor stem cells	stem cells than can become almost any cell or tissue with a preference for certain tissue types (i.e., mostly connective tissue with some blood cells)
PRP	platelet-rich plasma is not stem cells or matrix per se; it is the activated expression of a host of growth factors secreted by platelets that, in turn, act upon the tissue target, such as tendon or ligament
totipotent stem cells	stem cells (only present in blastocyst) that can become any cell or any tissue
umbilical cord blood stem cells	mostly hematopoietic stem cells that are especially suitable for becoming blood cells and immune regulators
umbilical cord stem cells	stem cells collected from the donated birth waste of healthy live newborns; umbilical cord stem cells are undifferentiated and to date have not been associated with oncogenesis nor do they themselves turn into cancer
umbilical cord wall stem cells	mostly mesenchymal stem cells that are especially suitable for becoming connective tissue

APPENDIX 2: NOTABLE DATES

1868 German scientist Valentin Häcker coins term "stammzelle" (German for stem cell)

1908 Russian scientist Alexander Maksimov and others use the term "stem cell" for their work in hematopoiesis

1963 McCulloch and Till (Ontario Cancer Institute Canada) illustrate the presence of stem cells in mouse bone marrow.

1968 First bone marrow transplant between siblings with severe comorbid immunodeficiency (SCID).

1974 First report on stem/progenitor cells in human cord blood.

1981 Gail Martin (UCSF) isolates stem cells from a mouse embryo.

1988 First successful cord blood transplant to regenerate blood and immune cells in Paris, France on a six-year-old boy suffering from Fanconi's Anemia (from identical twin sister).

1991 Dr. Arnold Caplan coins the term "mesenchymal stem cell."

1992 New York Blood Center establishes the first public CB bank.

1993 First unrelated allogeneic (UCB) transplant performed.

1996 First unrelated (allogeneic) cord blood transplant in adults.

1998 Netcord group is created in Canada to establish good practices in umbilical cord blood banking, and the first successful transplant is conducted to cure sickle cell anemia

2001 Research shows that cord blood is a suitable alternative to adults requiring a stem cell transplant.

2003 Successful stem cell treatment after stroke.

2006 Research increases in the use of cord blood to treat auto-immune diseases and brain disorders.

2011 Ministers of Health announce Canada's first national, publicly-funded umbilical cord blood bank managed by Canadian Blood Services.

2012 Clinical trial for autism treated with self-cord blood stem cells begins in Sutter Neuroscience Institute, Sacramento, California.

2012 It is estimated that more than 35,000 cord blood transplants have been performed worldwide

2015 Along with cord blood, Wharton's jelly and the cord lining have been explored as sources for mesenchymal stem cells (MSC), and had been studied *in vitro* (in a laboratory), in animal models, and in early-stage clinical trials for cardiovascular diseases, as well as neurological deficits, liver diseases, immune system diseases, diabetes, lung injury, kidney injury, and leukemia.

2017 Over a million stem cell transplants are recorded worldwide.

History develops quickly, and we are destined to see many advances and discoveries, clinical applications, and, of course, more specific regulations ahead of us. Health care historians will eventually systematize and streamline major milestones of stem cell history. I challenge them to do this sooner rather than later.

APPENDIX 3A:
EXAMPLES OF GROWTH-REGULATING FACTORS

Growth factors found in stem cells		
Paracrine factor	**Organ/disease**	**Function**
Ang1 and 2 (angiopoietins)	Heart, wound healing	Angiogenesis
bFGF (basic growth factor)	Heart, wound healing, bone, nervous system	Cardio protection, angiogenesis, granulation tissue formation, capillary formation, bone formation and repair, neuroprotection
BMP-4 (bone morphogenic protein)	Bone, nervous system	Determines NSC, NPC, bone formation and repair
BDNF, GDNF	Nervous system	Protects motor neurons, increased D neuron survival
IGF-1	Nervous system, heart	Protects motor neurons, cardio protection, angiogenesis, recruits progenitor cells, activates CSC
IL-7	Bone marrow	Supports hematopoiesis
MMPs (matrix metalloproteinase)	Heart, bone, cancer	Establishes ECF homeostasis, inhibits fibrosis, regulates bone ECM, tumor growth and migration
NGF	Nervous system	Increased D neuron survival, delineates the lineage specification for NSC and NPC
NT-3 (neurotrophin)	Nervous system	Survival and differentiation of existing and new neurons and synapses
TNF-alpha	Heart	Angiogenesis

APPENDIX 3B:
EXAMPLES OF IMMUNE-REGULATING FACTORS

Immune regulating factors found in stem cells[157]		
Paracrine factor	**Organ/disease**	**Function**
HGF	Immune system, heart, wound healing	Inhibits T-cell proliferation, cytokine production and cytotoxicity, recruits progenitor cells, activated cardiac stem cells, granulation tissue, capillaries formation
IDO (indoleamine 2,3 dioxygenase)	Immune system	Inhibits T – and NK cells, cytokine production and cytotoxicity, mediates T-cell apoptosis
IL-1	Immune system, heart	mediates T-cell proliferation, cardio protection, neurogenesis
IL-6	Immune system, bone marrow, cancer	Mediates T- and B-cell proliferation, protects dendrites and neutrophils, role in tumor growth and migration
TGF-beta	Immune system, heart, bone	Inhibits T- and NK-cell proliferation, cytokine production and cytotoxicity, inhibits fibrosis; bone formation and repair

*Please note reference #157 applies to Appendix 3A and Appendix 3B.

APPENDIX 4:
POST STEM CELL TREATMENT INSTRUCTIONS

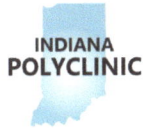

INDIANA POLYCLINIC
201 Pennsylvania Pkwy
Suite 200
Indianapolis, IN 46280
317-805-5500 (phone)
317-805-5501 (fax)

LIVE STEM CELLS
POST INFUSION/INJECTION INSTRUCTIONS

PATIENT COPY

Stem Cell Joint Injections

Heaviness in the body and flu-like sensations have been reported. This is normal, may last for 1-3 days and no action is needed.

> If the patient experiences fever or other severe unexpected complications, contact your doctor and/or seek emergency (ER) treatment.

Epidural/Intrathecal Stem Cell Administration

Heaviness in the body and flu-like sensations have been reported. This is normal, may last for 1-3 days and no action is needed.

> Fever, paralysis, severe headaches, seizures, and other severe symptoms are not expected - however, if the patient should experience any of these, they should immediately seek emergency (ER) treatment.

Stem Cell Joint Injections

Heaviness in the body and flu-like sensations have been reported. This is normal, may last for 1-3 days and no action is needed.

Swelling of the injected joint is common and can be severe. As long as there is no redness and fever, even significant swelling is OK. Gentle ice application and elevation of the extremity helps.

Pain in the injected joint is also common and can be severe. Without other symptoms, significant pain does not indicate that something is wrong.

> If the patient experiences fever or other severe unexpected complications, contact your doctor and/or seek emergency (ER) treatment.

For mild to moderate pain and swelling patients may use Tylenol alone. For severe pain, patients may need Tylenol 1000mg in combination with ibuprofen 800mg up to three times a day. The more swelling and pain, the more ibuprofen is needed. Sometimes the pain may be severe enough that a few doses of an opioid medication may be needed. Anti-inflammatory medications such as ibuprofen may negatively affect stem cells shortly after their introduction in the joint and, when possible, should be avoided.

Physical Therapy (PT) and exercise after Stem Cell joint treatments

Avoid high impact activities for about 3 months post-injection (such as running, etc.) PT sessions are recommended to be reduced in the strenuousness of the session by about 25% during the first 2 weeks and increase slowly over the course of about the next 8 weeks. If you lift weights, reduce the weight by about 25-50% depending on how heavy the weights were to start with (moderate weights - 25% / heavy weights - 50%) and increase over the course of 8 to 12 weeks.

Acupuncture and other alternative treatments after Stem Cells

Acupuncture is unlikely to impede stem cells and actually may enhance their function. The use of electro-acupuncture post stem cell treatment is controversial. Until more is known, it is probably better to avoid electro-acupuncture, moxibustion, or cupping for at least 2-3 weeks post stem cell treatment.

APPENDIX 5: CURRENT STEM CELL STUDIES

Stem Cell Studies		
Study Search Term	United States	Total
stem cells	2,610	5,249
mesenchymal stem cells	147	774
umbilical cord stem cells	59	228
umbilical cord blood stem cells	81	128

Source: ClinicalTrials.gov (accessed on August 24, 2019) - includes completed and withdrawn studies

ACKNOWLEDGMENTS

My deepest gratitude goes to the patients who underwent stem cell treatments and shared their experience with me. I must thank my friend, publisher, and stickler to English rules Paul Adams. Matt Jager, thank you, you are my deeply and deservingly respected editor. Thank you, Dr. Mark Erwin, of Notogen Inc., and the University of Toronto, for providing the invaluable critique of a cellular scientist; Dr. Eliott Spenser of Utah Cord Blood Bank, whose view on exosomes shaped my insight; Stu Bowes who applied a decisive push to dump me into the turbulent waters of stem cells; Dr. Ursula Jacob, my first stem cell teacher; Dr. Scheffer Tseng, whose innovation in stem cell science is impossible to overestimate; Lily Hills who helped me to come up with the name of this book; Anthony Gattone for his wisdom on religion; Indiana Polyclinic doctors Rachel Boggus and Brian Paquette who skillfully and successfully do every day what others would dream doing once in a lifetime. The endless animals who give their lives for us to know more about the world have to be profoundly thanked. And, of course, I am endlessly thankful to my family and friends to whom this little book is devoted.

INDEX

Endnotes

1   Adapted from Nathan and Ding. Cell, 140:871-882, 2010

2   Zimmerman A, Jyonouchi H, Comi A, et al. Cerebrospinal Fluid and Serum Markers of Inflammation in Autism, Pediatric Neurology, (Sept 2005);33(3):195-201

3   Bergin V, Gibney S, Drexhage H. Autoimmunity, Inflammation, and Psychosis: A Search for Peripheral Markers, Biological Psychiatry (February 2014);75(4):324-331

4   Miller A, Raison C. The role of inflammation in depression: from evolutionary imperative to modern treatment target . Nat Rev Immunol. January 2016; 16(1): 22–34.

5   Hwang SH., Kim MH., Yang IH et al., Analysis of cytokines in umbilical cord blood-derived multipotent stem cells. Biotechnology and Bioprocess Bioengineering. 2007,12:32-38

6   E. Soleymaninejadian, K. Pramanik, and E. Samadian, Immunomodulatory properties of mesenchymal stem cells: cytokines and factors. American Journal of Reproductive Immunology. 2012;67(1):1-8

7   Dvorak HF, Tumors: wounds that do not heal. Similarities between tumor stroma generation and wound healing N Engl J Med. 1986 Dec 25; 315(26):1650-9

8   Abbott JD, Huang Y, Liu D, Hickey R, et al. Stromal cell-derived factor-1alpha plays a critical role in stem cell recruitment to the heart after myocardial infarction but is not sufficient to induce homing in the absence of injury. Circulation. 2004 Nov 23; 110(21):3300-5.

9   Zhang HT, Fan J, Cai YQ, Zhao SJ, Xue S, Lin JH, Jiang XD, Xu RX. Human Wharton's jelly cells can be induced to differentiate into growth factor-secreting oligodendrocyte progenitor-like cells. Differentiation. 2010;79:15–20

10 Campard D, Lysy PA, Najimi M, Sokal EM. Native umbilical cord matrix stem cells express hepatic markers and differentiate into hepatocyte-like cells. Gastroenterology. 2008;134:833–848

11 Dellavalle A, Maroli G, Covarello D, Azzoni E, Innocenzi A, Perani L, et al. Pericytes resident in postnatal skeletal muscle differentiate into muscle fibres and generate satellite cells. Nat Commun. 2011;2:499.

12 Memorial Sloan Kettering Cancer Center. Allogeneic Stem Cell Transplant: A Guide for Patients & Caregivers, 2017

13 Jennifer Choi. Assimetric cell division: its implication for stem cells and cancer. February 24, 2017 Biol 312 @UNBC – Molecular cell physiology

14 Arutyunyan I, Elchaninov A, Makarov A, Fatkhudinov T. Umbilical Cord as Prospective Source for Mesenchymal Stem Cell-Based Therapy. Stem Cells International Volume 2016, Article ID 6901286

15 Andrew S. Rowlands et al. Am J Physiol Cell Physiol 2008;295:C1037-C1044

16 Marie-Luce VIGNAIS. Role of mesenchymal stem/stromal cells (MSCs) in the microenvironment. Model system: interactions between MSCs and cancer cells. Regulation of the energetic metabolism. INSERM U1183 "Cellules Souches, Plasticité Cellulaire, Médecine Régénératrice Et Immunothérapies"

17 https://phys.org/news/2015-04-age-discrimination-cell-division-stem-cells.html#jCp

18 Fong CY, Gauthaman K, Cheyyatraivendran S, Lin HD, Biswas A, Bongso A. Human umbilical cord Wharton's jelly stem cells and its conditioned medium support hematopoietic stem cell expansion ex vivo. J Cell Biochem. 2012;113:658–668

19 Guilherme V. Silva, Silvio Litovsky, Joao A.R. Assad ed al. Mesenchymal Stem Cells Differentiate into an Endothelial Phenotype, Enhance Vascular Density, and Improve Heart Function in a

Canine Chronic Ischemia Model. Circulation. 2005;111:150-156

20 Ning Yuan1, Wei Tian1, Lei Sun, et al., Neural stem cell transplantation in a double-layer collagen membrane with unequal pore sizes for spinal cord injury repair. Neural Regeneration Research. 2014; 9:10,1014-1019

21 Andrea Gärtner, Tiago Pereira, Raquel Gomes et al., Mesenchymal Stem Cells from Extra-Embryonic Tissues for Tissue Engineering – Regeneration of the Peripheral Nerve. "Advances in Biomaterials Science and Biomedical Applications" Chapter 18, March 27, 2013

22 Seaberg, R. M.; Van Der Kooy, D. "Stem and progenitor cells: The premature desertion of rigorous definitions." Trends in Neurosciences. 2003;26(3):125–131

23 Mason, John O.; Price, David J. "Building brains in a dish: Prospects for growing cerebral organoids from stem cells." Neuroscience. 2016; 334: 105–118

24 Bhartiya, D. Pluripotent Stem Cells in Adult Tissues: Struggling To Be Acknowledged Over Two Decades. Stem Cell Rev and Rep (2017) pp 1-12

25 Marks, P. W., Witten, C. M., & Califf, R. M. Clarifying stem-cell therapy's benefits and risks. The New England Journal of Medicine, 2017; 376(11), 1007–1009

26 Singer NG, Caplan AI. Mesenchymal stem cells: mechanisms of inflammation. Annu Rev Pathol. 2011;6:457–78

27 Caplan AI. Mesenchymal stem cells. J Orthop Res. 1991;9:641–50

28 Volarevic V. et al., Bio-Factors, 2018, in press

29 Gnecchi M, Melo LG. Bone marrow-derived mesenchymal stem cells: isolation, expansion, characterization, viral transduction, and production of conditioned medium. Methods Mol Biol. 2009;482:281–294

30 Zhang X, Hirai M, Cantero S, Ciubotariu R, et al. Isolation and characterization of mesenchymal stem cells from human umbilical cord blood: reevaluation of critical factors for successful isolation and high ability to proliferate and differentiate to chondrocytes as compared to mesenchymal stem cells from bone marrow and adipose tissue. J Cell Biochem. 2011;112:1206–1218.

31 Gimble J, Katz A, Bunnel B. Adipose-Derived Stem Cells for Regenerative Medicine. Circulation Research. 2007;100:1249-1260

32 Da Silva Meirelles L, Chagastelles PC, Nardi NB. Mesenchymal stem cells reside in virtually all post-natal organs and tissues. J Cell Sci 2006; 119: 2204–2213.

33 Anker, P.S., Scherjon, S.A., Kleijburg-van der Keur, C., et al. (2003) Amniotic fluid as a novel source of mesenchymal stem cells for therapeutic transplantation. Blood 102, 1548–1549

34 Sessarego N, Parodi A, Podesta` M, Benvenuto F, Mogni M, Raviolo V et al. Multipotent mesenchymal stromal cells from amniotic fluid: solid perspectives for clinical application. Haematologica 2008; 93:339–346.

35 Batsali AK, Kastrinaki MC, Papadaki HA, Pontikoglou C. Mesenchymal stem cells derived from Wharton's Jelly of the umbilical cord: biological properties and emerging clinical applications. Current stem cell research & therapy. 2013; 8: 144-155

36 Ishige I, Nagamura-Inoue T, Honda MJ, Harnprasopwat R, Kido M, Sugimoto M, Nakauchi H, Tojo A. Comparison of mesenchymal stem cells derived from arterial, venous, and Wharton's jelly explants of human umbilical cord. Int J Hematol. 2009;90:261–269

37 X.-J. Liang, X.-J. Chen, D.-H. Yang, S.-M. Huang, G.-D. Sun, and Y.-P. Chen, "Differentiation of human umbilical cord mesenchymal stem cells into hepatocyte-like cells by hTERT gene transfection in vitro," Cell Biology International, vol. 36, no. 2, pp. 215–221, 2012

38 Serakinci N, Graakjaer J, Kolvraa S. Telomere stability and telomerase in mesenchymal stem cells. Biochimie. 2008; 90: 33-40

39 Tollervey JR, Lunyak VV. Adult stem cells: simply a tool for regenerative medicine or an addi-

tional piece in the puzzle of human aging? Cell Cycle 2011; 10: 4173–4176.

40 Pipes BL, Tsang T, Peng SX, et al. Telomere length changes after umbilical cord blood transplant. Transfusion. 2006 Jun;46(6):1038-43

41 Mueller SM, Glowacki J. Age-related decline in the osteogenic potential of human bone marrow cells cultured in three-dimensional collagen sponges. J Cell Biochem. 2001;82:583–590

42 Campisi J, Cancer, aging, and cellular senescence. In Vivo. 2000 Jan-Feb; 14(1):183-8

43 Juhyun Oh, Yang David Lee et al. Stem cell aging: mechanisms, regulators and therapeutic opportunities. Nat Med. 2014 Aug 6; 20(8): 870–880.

44 Kern S, Eichler H, Stoeve J, Klüter H, Bieback K. Comparative analysis of mesenchymal stem cells from bone marrow, umbilical cord blood, or adipose tissue. Stem cells. 2006; 24: 1294-1301.

45 Arirachakaran A, Sukthuayat A, Sisayanarane T, et al. Platelet-rich plasma versus autologous blood versus steroid injection in lateral epicondylitis: a systematic review and network meta-analysis. J Orthop Traumatol. 2016 Jun; 17(2):101-12.

46 Foster TE, Puskas BL, Mandelbaum BR, Gerhardt MB, Rodeo SA. "Platelet-rich plasma: from basic science to clinical applications." Am J Sports Med. 2009; 37 (11): 2259–72

47 Frautschi, RS; Hashem, AM; Halasa, B; Cakmakoglu, C; Zins, JE (1 March 2017). "Current Evidence for Clinical Efficacy of Platelet Rich Plasma in Aesthetic Surgery: A Systematic Review.". Aesthetic surgery journal. 37 (3): 353–362

48 Catlin S, Busque L, Gaile R at al. (Aril 2011) The replication of human hematopoietic stem cells in vitro. Blood, 117(17):4460-66

49 Murphy MB1, Blashki D, Buchanan RM Adult and umbilical cord blood-derived platelet-rich plasma for mesenchymal stem cell proliferation, chemotaxis, and cryo-preservation. Biomaterials. 2012 Jul;33(21):5308-16

50 Park EH, White GA, Tieber LM. Mechanisms of injury and emergency care of acute spinal cord injury in dogs and cats. J Vet Emerg Crit Care (San Antonio). 2012;22(2):160-178.

51 Godwin EE, Young NJ, Dudhia J, Beamish IC, Smith RK. Implantation of bone marrow-derived mesenchymal stem cells demonstrates improved outcome in horses with overstrain injury of the superficial digital flexor tendon. Equine Vet J. 2012;44(1):25-32.

52 Cuervo B, Rubio M, Sopena J, et al. Hip osteoarthritis in dogs: a randomized study using mesenchymal stem cells from adipose tissue and plasma rich in growth factors. Int J Mol Sci. 2014;15(8):13437-13460.

53 Harman R, Carlson K, Gaynor J, et al. A prospective, randomized, masked, and placebo-controlled efficacy study of intraarticular allogeneic adipose stem cells for the treatment of osteoarthritis in dogs. Front Vet Sci. 2016 Sep 16;3:81.

54 Beerts C, Suls M, Broeckx SY, et al. Tenogenically induced allogeneic peripheral blood mesenchymal stem cells in allogeneic platelet-rich plasma: 2-year follow-up after tendon or ligament treatment in horses. Front Vet Sci. 2017;4:158.

55 Van Loon VJ, Scheffer CJ, Genn HJ, Hoogendoom AC, Greve JW. Clinical follow-up of horses treated with allogeneic equine mesenchymal stem cells derived from umbilical cord blood for different tendon and ligament disorders. Vet Q. 2014;34(2):92-97.

56 Herberts CA1, Kwa MS, Hermsen HP Risk factors in the development of stem cell therapy. J.Transl. Med. 2011;9:29

57 Marks, P. W., Witten, C. M., & Califf, R. M. Clarifying stem-cell therapy's benefits and risks. The New England Journal of Medicine, 2017; 376(11), 1007–1009

58 Berkowitz AL et al. New England Journal of Medicine 2016 Jul 14;375(2):196-8

59 Rosemann A (Dec 2014). "Why regenerative stem cell medicine progresses slower than expect-

ed." J Cell Biochem. 115 (12): 2073–76

60 https://www.ecfr.gov/cgi-bin/retrieveECFR?gp=&SID=ff69887f399bdceb2b1f8ddaef-4d579e&mc=true&n=pt21.8.1271&r=PART&ty=HTML#se21.8.1271_145

61 https://www.fda.gov/news-events/press-announcements/fda-puts-company-notice-market-ing-unapproved-stem-cell-products-treating-serious-conditions

62 Thirumala, S., Goebel, W.S. and Woods, E.J. (2009) Clinical grade adult stem cell banking. Organogenesis 5, 143–154

63 Gruen L, Grabel L. Concise review: scientific and ethical roadblocks to human embryonic stem cell therapy. Stem Cells 2006;24(10):2162–2169.

64 Saha P, Sharma S, Korutla L et al. Circulating exosomes derived from transplanted progenitor cells aid the functional recovery of ischemic myocardium. Science Translational Medicine 2019 May 22 ; 11 (493), eaau1168

65 Zambelli A, Poggi G, Da Prada G, et al.,(1998) Clinical toxicity of cryopreserved circulating progenitor cells infusion. Anticancer Res 18:4705–8.

66 Bissoyi A, Pramanik K. Role of the apoptosis pathway in cryopreservation-induced cell death in mesenchymal stem cells derived from umbilical cord blood. Biopreserv Biobank 2014;12:246-254

67 Yuan C, Gao J, Guo J, et al. (2014) Dimethyl Sulfoxide Damages Mitochondrial, Integrity and Membrane Potential in Cultured Astrocytes. PLoS ONE 9(9): e107447.

68 Quintanar N., Patel R., Jones C., Importance of development of non-DMSO containing preservatives Progenokine® Process and the effects of Cellular Viability from Umbilical Cord Blood Adherent Cells. Department of Research and Development, Burst Biologics, 2017

69 Holm F, Stro S, Inzunz J. (March 2010), An effective serum- and xeno-free chemically defined freezing procedure for human embryonic and induced pluripotent stem cells Reproduct Biol. 25 (5): 1271–79, 201

70 Weng JY, Du X, Geng SX, Peng YW, et al. Mesenchymal stem cell as salvage treatment for refractory chronic GVHD. Bone Marrow Transplant. 2010;45:1732–1740

71 Le Blanc K, Frassoni F, Ball L, et al. Mesenchymal stem cells for treatment of steroid-resistant, severe, acute graft-versus-host disease: a Phase II study. Lancet 2008;371(9624):1579–1586.

72 Ringden O, Uzunel M, Rasmusson I, et al. Mesenchymal stem cells for treatment of therapy-resistant graft-versus-host disease. Transplantation 2006;81(10):1390–1397.

73 See Bernaudin F et al., Long-term results of related myeloablative stem-cell transplantation to cure sickle cell disease. Blood. 2007;110:2749-2756. "Hematopoietic stem cell transplantation (HSCT) is the only curative therapy for sickle cell disease."

74 Feng J, Mantesso A, De Bari C, Nishiyama A, Sharpe PT. Dual origin of mesenchymal stem cells contributing to organ growth and repair. Proc Natl Acad Sci U S A. 2011;108:6503–8.

75 Fufaeva E, Semenova J, Semenova N, Sidorin S. Dynamics of high mental function recovery in children after severe traumatic brain injury having umbilical cord blood cells therapy. Brain Inj. 2012;26:688-689

76 DMEnnis J, Götherström C, Le Blanc K, Davies JE. In vitro immunologic properties of human umbilical cord perivascular cells. Cytotherapy. 2008;10:174–181

77 Weiss ML, Anderson C, Medicetty S, et al. Immune properties of human umbilical cord Wharton's jelly-derived cells. Stem Cells. 2008;26:2865–2874

78 Figueroa, F.F., Carri´on, F., Villanueva, S. and Khoury, M. (2012) Mesenchymal Stem Cell treatment for autoimmune diseases: a critical review. Biol. Res. 45, 269–77

79 Furlani D, Ugurlucan M, Ong L, Bieback K, Pittermann E, Westien I, et al. Is the intravascular administration of mesenchymal stem cells safe? Mesenchymal stem cells and intravital micros-

copy. Microvascular Research. 2009; 77: 370-376

80   Krasnodembskaya A, Samarani G, Song Y, Zhuo H, Su X, et al. (2012) Human mesenchymal stem cells reduce mortality and bacteremia in gram-negative sepsis in mice in part by enhancing the phagocytic activity of blood monocytes. Am J Physiol Lung Cell Mol Physiol 302: L1003–1013

81   Krasnodembskaya A, Song Y, Fang X, Gupta N, Serikov V, et al. (2010) Antibacterial effect of human mesenchymal stem cells is mediated in part from secretion of the antimicrobial peptide LL-37. Stem Cells 28: 2229–2238.

82   Xiaojia Huang, Kai Sun1, Yidan D. Zhao, et al., Human CD34+ Progenitor Cells Freshly Isolated from Umbilical Cord Blood Attenuate Inflammatory Lung Injury following LPS Challenge PLOS ONE February 2014;9(2)

83   Pierro M, Ionescu L, Montemurro T, Vadivel A, Weissmann G, et al. (2013) Short-term, long-term and paracrine effect of human umbilical cord-derived stem cells in lung injury prevention and repair in experimental bronchopulmonary dysplasia. Thorax 68: 475–484.

84   Mao Q, Chu S, Ghanta S, Padbury JF, De Paepe ME (2013) Ex vivo expanded human cord blood-derived hematopoietic progenitor cells induce lung growth and alveolarization in injured newborn lungs. Respir Res 14: 37.

85   Nakajima H, Uchida K, Guerrero AR, Watanabe S, Sugita D, Takeura N et al. Transplantation of mesenchymal stem cells promotes an alternative pathway of macrophage activation and functional recovery after spinal cord injury. J Neurotrauma 2012; 29: 1614–1625

86   Park JH, Kim DY, Sung IY, Choi GH, Jeon MH, Kim KK et al. Long-term results of spinal cord injury therapy using mesenchymal stem cells derived from bone marrow in humans. Neurosurgery 2012; 70: 1238–1247.

87   Chevalier X. Intraarticular treatments for osteoarthritis: new perspectives. Curr Drug Targets. 2010 May;11(5):546-60. Review

88   John A. Anderson, Dianne Little, Alison P. Toth, et al. Stem Cell Therapies for Knee Cartilage Repair The American Journal of Sports Medicine PreView, November 12, 2013

89   Shin Y-S, JungRo Yoon J-R, KimIntra H-S, et al. Articular Injection of Bone MarrowDerived Mesenchymal Stem Cells Leading to Better Clinical Outcomes without Difference in MRI Outcomes from Baseline in Patients with Knee Osteoarthritis Knee Surg Relat Res 2018;30(3):206-214

90   Gruber HE. Hanley ENJ. Recent advances in disc cell biology. Spine 2003; 28: 186–193

91   Ganey T, Hutton WC, Moseley T, Hedrick M, Meisel H-J. Intervertebral disc repair using adipose tissue-derived stem and regenerative cells: experiments in a canine model. Spine 2009; 34: 2297–2304.

92   Erwin WM , Islam D , Eftekarpour E, at al. Intervertebral Disc-Derived Stem Cells Implications for Regenerative Medicine and Neural Repair. SPINE 2013;38(3):211–216

93   www.DiscGenics.com

94   Zebardast N, Lickorish D, Davies JE. Human umbilical cord perivascular cells (HUCPVC): A mesenchymal cell source for dermal wound healing. Organogenesis. 2010;6:197–203

95   Conconi MT, Burra P, Di Liddo R, Calore C, Turetta M, Bellini S, Bo P, Nussdorfer GG, Parnigotto PP. CD105(+) cells from Wharton's jelly show in vitro and in vivo myogenic differentiative potential. Int J Mol Med. 2006;18:1089–1096

96   Chaudhuri B, Pramanik K. Key aspects of the mesenchymal stem cells (MSCs) in tissue engineering for in vitro skeletal muscle regeneration. Biotechnol Mol Biol Rev 2012; 7: 5–15

97   Chen L, Tredget EE, Wu PYG, Wu Y. Paracrine factors of mesenchymal stem cells recruit macrophages and endothelial lineage cells and enhance wound healing. PLoS One 2008; 3: e1886

98   Parekkadan B, Milwid JM. Mesenchymal stem cells as therapeutics. Annu Rev Biomed Eng 2010; 12: 87–117

99   Uysal AC, et al. Differentiation of adipose-derived stem cells for tendon repair. Methods Mol. Biol. 2011;702:443-51.

100   Doorn J, van de Peppel J, van Leeuwen JPTM, Groen N, van Blitterswijk CA, de Boer J. Pro-osteogenic trophic effects by PKA activation in human mesenchymal stromal cells. Biomaterials 2011; 32: 6089–6098.

101   Parekkadan B, Milwid JM. Mesenchymal stem cells as therapeutics. Annu Rev Biomed Eng 2010; 12: 87–117

102   Mohanty ST, Bellantuono I. Intra-femoral injection of human mesenchymal stem cells. Methods Mol Biol. 2013;976:131–41.

103   Kawamoto A, Tkebuchava T, Yamaguchi J, Nishimura H, Yoon YS, et al. Intramyocardial transplantation of autologous endothelial progenitor cells for therapeutic neovascularization of myocardial ischemia. Circulation 2003;107: 461–468.

104   Assmus B, Schachinger V, Teupe C, Britten M, Lehmann R, et al. Transplantation of Progenitor Cells and Regeneration Enhancement in Acute Myocardial Infarction (TOPCARE-AMI). Circulation 2002; 106: 3009–3017.

105   Cselenya´k A, Pankotai E, Horva´th EM, Kiss L, Lacza Z. Mesenchymal stem cells rescue cardiomyoblasts from cell death in an in vitro ischemia model via direct cell-to-cell connections. BMC Cell Biol 2010; 11: 29.

106   Lipinski MJ, Luger D, Epstein SE. Mesenchymal Stem Cell Therapy for the Treatment of Heart Failure Caused by Ischemic or Non-ischemic Cardiomyopathy: Immunosuppression and Its Implications. Handb Exp Pharmacol. 2017;243:329-353

107   www.mesoblast.com

108   Shyu WC, Lin SZ, Chiang MF, Su CY, Li H Intracerebral peripheral blood stem cell (CD34+) implantation induces neuroplasticity by enhancing beta1 integrin-mediated angiogenesis in chronic stroke rats. J Neurosci 2006;26: 3444–3453

109   Muir KW, Sinden J, Miljan E, Dunn L. Intracranial delivery of stem cells. Transl Stroke Res. 2011 Sep;2(3):266-71

110   Woodworth C, Jenkins G, Barron J at al. Intramedullary cervical spinal mass after stem cell transplantation using an olfactory mucosal cell autograft CMAJ July 08, 2019 191 (27) E761-E764

111   Weiss JN, Levy S, Malkin A. Stem Cell Ophthalmology Treatment Study (SCOTS) for retinal and optic nerve diseases: a preliminary report. Neural Regen Res 2015; 10:982-8;

112   Weiss JN, Levy S, Benes SC. Stem Cell Ophthalmology Treatment Study (SCOTS) for retinal and optic nerve diseases: a case report of improvement in relapsing auto-immune optic neuropathy. Neural Regen Res 2015; 10:1507-15.

113   Labrador-Velandia S, Alonso-Alonso ML, Alvarez-Sanchez S, et al. , Mesenchymal stem cell therapy in retinal and optic nerve diseases: An update of clinical trials. World J Stem Cells. 2016 Nov 26;8(11):376-383

114   Zhang C., Yang SJ, Wen Q. et al. Human-derived normal mesenchymal stem/stromal cells in anticancer therapies Journal of Cancer 2017; 8(1): 85-96

115   Zhao W, Ren G, Zhang L, et al. Efficacy of mesenchymal stem cells derived from human adipose tissue in inhibition of hepatocellular carcinoma cells in vitro. Cancer Biother Radiopharm. 2012; 27: 606-13.

116   Matsuzuka T, Rachakatla RS, Doi C, et al. Human umbilical cord matrix-derived stem cells expressing interferon-β gene significantly attenuate bronchioloalveolar carcinoma xenografts in SCID mice. Lung Cancer. 2010; 70: 28-36

117   Goldstein RH, Reagan MR, Anderson K, et al. Human bone marrow-derived MSCs can home to

orthotopic breast cancer tumors and promote bone metastasis. Cancer Res. 2010; 70

118 Chu Y, Tang H, Guo Y, et al. Adipose-derived mesenchymal stem cells promote cell proliferation and invasion of epithelial ovarian cancer. Exp Cell Res. 2015; 337: 16-27.

119 Lalu MM, McIntyre L, Pugliese C, et al. Safety of cell therapy with mesenchymal stromal cells (SafeCell): a systematic review and meta-analysis of clinical trials. PLoS One. 2012; 7: e47559.

120 Dong L, Pu Y, Zhang L, et al. Human umbilical cord mesenchymal stem cell-derived extracellular vesicles promote lung adenocarcinoma growth by transferring miR-410 Cell Death and Disease (2018) 9:218

121 Wu S, Ju GQ, Du T. et al. Microvesicles derived from human umbilical cord Wharton's jelly mesenchymal stem cells attenuate bladder tumor cell growth in vitro and in vivo. PLoS ONE 8, e61366 (2013).

122 Vickers R, Karsten E, Flood J, Lilischkis R, A preliminary report on stem cell therapy for neuropathic pain in humans Journal of Pain Research 2014;7: 255–263

123 Vallejo R, Tilley DM, Vogel L, Benyamin R. The role of glia and the immune system in the development and maintenance of neuropathic pain. Pain Pract. 2010;10(3):167–184.

124 Guo W, Wang H, Zou S, et al. Bone marrow stromal cells produce long-term pain relief in rat models of persistent pain. Stem Cells. 2011;29(8):1294–1303.

125 Sacerdote P, Niada S, Franchi S, et al. Systemic administration of human adipose-derived stem cells reverts nociceptive hypersensitivity in an experimental model of neuropathy. Stem Cells Dev. 2013;22(8):1252–1263.

126 Franchi S, Valsecchi AE, Borsani E, et al. Intravenous neural stem cells abolish nociceptive hypersensitivity and trigger nerve regeneration in experimental neuropathy. Pain. 2012;153(4):850–861.

127 https://www.intechopen.com/books/regenerative-medicine-and-tissue-engineering/dental-related-stem-cells-and-their-potential-in-regenerative-medicine

128 Nokhbatolfoghahaei H, Rad MR, Khani MM, et al., Application of bioreactors to improve functionality of bone tissue engineering constructs: A systematic review. Curr Stem Cell Res Ther. 2017 Aug 21

129 Mangione F, EzEldeen M, Bardet C, et al. Implanted Dental Pulp Cells Fail to Induce Regeneration in Partial Pulpotomies. J Dent Res. 2017 Aug 1

130 Bajestan MN, Rajan A, Edwards SP, et al. Stem cell therapy for reconstruction of alveolar cleft and trauma defects in adults: A randomized controlled, clinical trial. Clin Implant Dent Relat Res. 2017 Jun 28

131 Tobita M, et al. Periodontal tissue regeneration with adipose-derived stem cells. Tissue Eng. Part A. 2008;14(6):945-953.

132 Wu DC, Goldman MP. A Prospective, Randomized, Double-blind, Split-face Clinical Trial Comparing the Efficacy of Two Topical Human Growth Factors for the Rejuvenation of the Aging Face. J Clin Aesthet Dermatol. 2017 May;10(5):31-35

133 Ji J, Ho BS, Qian G, Xie XM, Bigliardi PL, Bigliardi-Qi MAging in hair follicle stem cells and niche microenvironment. J Dermatol. 2017 Jun 8

134 Deng W, et al. Mesenchymal stem cells regenerate skin tissue. Tissue Engineering. 2005;11:110-9.

135 Mansilla, E et al., A Rat Treated with Mesenchymal Stem Cells Lives to 44 Months of Age. Rejuvenation Res. 2016 Aug 1; 19(4): 318–321.

136 Segel M, Neumann BM, Hill M, et al. Niche stiffness underlies the ageing of central nervous system progenitor cells Nature (August 14, 2019)

137 Goodell, M. A. & Rando, T. A. Stem cells and healthy aging. Science (2015)350, 1199–1204

138 Geissler S, Textor M, Kuhnisch J, Konnig D, Klein O, et al. (2012) Functional comparison of chronological and in vitro aging: differential role of the cytoskeleton and mitochondria in mesenchymal stromal cells. PLoS One 7: e52700.

139 Izadpanah R, Kaushal D, Kriedt C, Tsien F, Patel B, et al. (2008) Long-term in vitro expansion alters the biology of adult mesenchymal stem cells. Cancer Res 68: 4229–4238.

140 Akita S, Hayashida K, Takaki S, et al. The neck burn scar contracture: a concept of effective treatment. Burns Trauma. 2017 Jul 13;5:22

141 Zhao B, Zhang Y, Han S, Zhang W et al., Exosomes derived from human amniotic epithelial cells accelerate wound healing and inhibit scar formation. J Mol Histol. 2017 Apr;48(2):121-132

142 Spiekman M, van Dongen JA, Willemsen JC et al. The power of fat and its adipose-derived stromal cells: emerging concepts for fibrotic scar treatment. J Tissue Eng Regen Med. 2017 Feb 3

143 Sorg H, Tilkorn DJ, Hager S, Hauser J, Skin Wound Healing: An Update on the Current Knowledge and Concepts. Eur Surg Res. 2017;58(1-2):81-94

144 Papanna et al. Cryopreserved Human Umbilical Cord Patch for In-utero Myeloschisis Repair. Obstet Gynecol, 128:325-30, 2016

145 Courtesy Scheffer Tseng, MD

146 Fufaeva E, Semenova J, Semenova N, Sidorin S. Dynamics of high mental function recovery in children after severe traumatic brain injury having umbilical cord blood cells therapy. Brain Inj. 2012;26:688-689

147 Dawson G, Sun L.M., Davlantis K., et al., Autologous Cord Blood Infusions Are Safe and Feasible in Young Children with Autism Spectrum Disorder: Results of a Single-Center Phase I Open-Label Trial. Stem Cells Translational Medicine. 2017;6:1332–1339

148 Shahaduzzaman M, Golden JE, Green S, et al. A single administration of human umbilical cord blood T cells produces longlasting effects in the aging hippocampus. Age (Dordr) 2013;35:2071–2087.

149 Cotten CM, Murtha AP, Goldberg RN et al. Promising Therapies for Alzheimer's Disease.

150 Confaloni A, Tosto G, Tata AM. Curr Pharm Des. 2016;22(14):2050-6 Feasibility of autologous cord blood cells for infants with hypoxic-ischemic encephalopathy. J Pediatr 2014;164:973–979.e1.

151 Yedy I, Ezquer F, Quintanilla ME at al. Intracerebral Stem Cell Administration Inhibits Relapse-like Alcohol Drinking in Rats. Alcohol and Alcoholism, January 2017;52(1): 1–4

152 https://clinicaltrials.gov/ct2/show/NCT01534624

153 Gratwohl A et al., One million hematopoietic stem-cell transplants: a retrospective observational study, Lancet Haematology 2, e91-e100, March 2015

154 Ballen KK, Gluckman E, Broxmeyer HE, Umbilical cord blood transplantation: the first 25 years and beyond, Blood. 122:491-498, 2013

155 Press release: "The Lancet Hematology: Experts warn of stem cell underuse as transplants reach 1 million worldwide" (Feb 26, 2016) http://www.eurekalert.org/pub_releases/2015-02/tl-tlh022515.php,

156 Zhang J, Huang X, Wang H, Liu X, Zhang T, Wang Y, Hu D. The challenges and promises of allogeneic mesenchymal stem cells for use as a cell-based therapy. Stem Cell Res Ther. 2015 Dec 1;6:234. Review

157 Baraniak P., McDevitt T., Stem cell paracrine action and tissue regeneration Regen Med 2010 Jan; 5(1):121-143

www.ingramcontent.com/pod-product-compliance
Lightning Source LLC
Chambersburg PA
CBHW060815270326
41930CB00002B/47